Also by Natalia Rose:

The Raw Food Detox Diet

Raw Food Life Force Energy

FOR OUR COSMIC BODY:

MAY WE COME TO PERCEIVE IT WITH EAGLE VISION!

This book is written as a source of information only. The information contained in this book should by no means be considered a substitute for the advice of a qualified medical professional, who should always be consulted before beginning any new diet or other health program. The author expressly disclaims responsibility for any adverse effects arising from the use or application of the information contained herein.

Library of Congress Cataloging-in-Publication Data
Rose, Natalia
    The New Energy Body: Discover a Hidden Source of Energy That Will Amaze You/ Natalia Rose – 1st edition.

ACKNOWLEDGEMENTS

I have had the benefit of the most marvelous teachers, healers and guides gifting me with the very insights I needed to pass through the life-enhancing doorways this book reflects. I give endless gratitude to Amorah Quan Yin, Almine Barton, Lee Harris, Story Waters, Nicola Robins and Ormungandr Melchizedek – you five helped catapult me out of my previously perceived limitations through your inspirational words and meditations. You have my love, praise and gratitude.

Tremendous thanks also to forward thinking scientists: Bruce Tainio, Bruce Lipton, Gregg Braden, Itzak Bentov, David Bohm, Dr. Candace Pert, Gary Zukav, Dr. Masaru Emoto, Drunvalo Melchizedek and William Tiller who gave me the insights I needed to take my hunches to the next level! You all lived your part to enlighten and ready the world for the mass enlightenment to come.

My dearest Lawrence, what do I say to the man I have loved my entire life who has given me the space and comforts to completely be myself despite all that required? You are a beacon of perfect masculine balance. I love you. I treasure you. I am yours.

My beloved daughter, Alexandra Thandi and my boy, Tommy Slade, you are my kindred spirits. I hope you both always feel your abundant love is joyfully received and reflected back million-fold. My Mother, Rita Barrett and my brother, Roman Barrett: you have nurtured my growth in greater ways than you will ever know. I love you, cherish you and thank you.

I could not have accomplished this project without the critical support, guidance and insights from my beloved friends, Birgin Juen, Angela Osborne-Coucher, Judith Regan, Batya Lahav, Samah Fares and Jad Itani.

Finally, a very special thank you to Gerardo Somoza for capturing the lively photo on the cover and to my design team: Tim Roberts and George Roberts of <u>Crucialnetworking.com</u> for their commitment to this project and my website.

CONTENTS

ON A PERSONAL NOTE

When I started down this path I never dreamed how far it would take me. All I was looking for 10 years ago was a more attractive, better functioning physicality. I just wanted to be released from the prison of my "wobbly bits," chronic bronchitis, depression and skin blemishes. Ordinarily, this in and of itself should have been more than enough to satisfy! But once I achieved all I desired on a physical level, I was reawakened to another quest – the great mystery of our existence – something I chalked up to being imponderable since I was six years old and told that our life is and will always remain a mystery. "That's God's plan," I was sternly rebuked, "and we don't need to understand it we simply need to revere it." So why was I bringing it up again now at 32? Obedience never was a strong suit.

The real reason, I now know is that my role is one of harvesting. I enjoy going out and pounding down the doors of truth for the answers that I know my fellow human family also seeks. I have had the distinct opportunity (for which I am deeply grateful) of being able to harvest and then distill this information into a form that is easily digestible for others.

I am not a scientist or a doctor. I am just a layperson with the ambition of fully understanding my life. Right or wrong, I feel that my desire to understand is not unlike everyone else's. I have been told that most people are not interested in understanding truths about their lives – particularly if doing so requires risking their illusions of safety. I respectfully disagree. I think that people DO care and deeply desire to understand why they are here, what they are really made of, what their purpose is and how they can live enriching lives and know themselves and their world with ever-expanding clarity.

The trouble is that the common ways of living have trained us to participate in the "assembly line" mentality by which the Western world is organized. We Westerners are placed on a conveyor belt of consumption and programming from the moment we emerge from the womb. Most people remain in that "factory" mentality throughout their lives, consuming what they are told to consume and swallowing questions or emotions that might disrupt the illusion of control around them until they are finally sent out to pasture.

For all of you who are no longer interested in stepping in line with the old, fruitless way I offer you another way of perceiving your lives, your innate power, your future, your health and your panoramic perspective of life. This is the way of The New Energy Body!

I'm here to say that our lives are not a mystery destined to remain hidden from us. If that were really the case, the finger print of life would not be on every living thing as it is. What is remarkable is that despite how obvious the language of life is and the answers are that appear in every iota of our lives, we still remain blind to them. Once you start to see these answers you will marvel at why and how you didn't see them all before.

In addition to the truths that were revealed through my quest, this book is also the result of accumulated experiences I have enjoyed as a direct result of detoxifying my body through the principles in my first book, *The Raw Food Detox Diet* and raising my Life Force Energy quotient through the insights of my

second book, *Raw Food Life Force Energy*. What happened as a result of transforming my physicality was that every aspect of my inner and outer life started unfolding more beautifully and harmoniously with every new day. It seemed that through these practices, I ignited a fire of inner power and lasting serenity that became self sustaining.

Of course, I could not simply rest on my "blissed-out" laurels and hoard paradise for myself. I had to fully understand what was driving this state in me both in layman's terms and scientifically so that I could share it. But one thing was clear. What I thought were our human limitations before dramatically expanded! In uncovering my own essence, I learned the tools to help anyone to uncover *their* own essence. While this project has a very wide scope, listen for the truths that you are ready to apply. There is time to absorb it all.

The power of this information is not, as I have learned, in its immediate apprehension and application, but rather in the ring of truth it carries which your body and heart will respond to as you are ready.

Uncovering the truths I sought has been the most fun and most rewarding ride of my life. That's saying a lot because after uncovering the secrets of an ideal *physical* existence I didn't think life could get any better. But hold on tight because what lies ahead will change the way you see yourself and your potential forever. Life is about to go from black and white to Technicolor!

My aim is to help you see that you are a living kingdom inside and out that is pure majesty and splendor. You already hold all the keys to that kingdom but I will help show you how to access them. It's not that you lack the tools to find them on your own; it's just that the modern way of living has interfered with your natural abilities. We will remedy this; you will unlock your palace doors and lower the drawbridge for your royal homecoming!

Many of you reading this may be aligned with a specific spiritual path. This is common to those seeking this type of knowledge. What you will find is that every great spiritual tradition has hidden within it the same core truths that we will be illuminating here. All are welcome with open mind and open heart. Those who truly seek will indeed find their answers.

There is a lot at play here – much more than meets the eye and it is the aim of this work to address readers at every stage. The goal is simply to make you more conscious than you were before. This can happen in big and small ways and we should rejoice every time it happens – to whatever extent it occurs.

Some of you will stick close to the obvious points. Others of you will go a little deeper and let your intuition take you into new a territory of thinking. Still others of you will be able to see the ultimate picture unfolding and carry the concepts into all aspects of your perspectives – your inner world and your outer world. I welcome, encourage and delight with each of you!

THE NEW BEAUTY

"Your body is the harp of your soul. It is yours to bring forth sweet music or confused sounds." – Kahlil Gibran

As an avid observer of trends and trend predictions, I have noted a significant shift in what we find beautiful in our culture. Instead of continuing to value youth for the sake of youth and flawlessness for the sake of flawlessness, I find that as people awaken they are starting to look less for commonly held ideals of perfection in terms of external beauty and more for beauty that shines from within and manifests without in the form of a fresh, natural glow. Personal authenticity is growing more valuable while plastic perfection is being seen for the illusion that it is.

Any good art designer or plastic surgeon can produce a perfect image. That's old hat. The new beauty (you might say it is the "original beauty") is one that shines from within – not just some image of commonly accepted perfection that we are conditioned to call "beauty."   Clarity and love are the new beauty and, over time, those who embody unconditional love and increase the love-light within themselves will be seen to be (and actually will be) physically more attractive. Plastic surgery, chemicals and the like place more density and poison in our being. With your New Energy Body you will naturally blossom into greater visual beauty too!

I already see my contemporaries preferring to be around others that are pure of purpose and of spirit. The people that I know of that are leaders and think for themselves are choosing friends, dates and mates who embody this inner beauty first; beauty for the sake of beauty is not "de rigeur" and will eventually be recognized as meaningless as more and more people awaken to the illusion of the old beauty. People want to be around other people that make them feel good and are good to others. I mention this specifically because so many of my readers are in search of ways to become more attractive and may have been drawn to this book in an attempt to improve their physical appearance. That will come; I can assure you – for the rejuvenation of the body, the heart and your hidden energy source are all inexorably connected.

An authentic glow, the result of dropping old patterns, aggression and fears and truly being oneself is the new "hot." Are you ready to sizzle? If not, definitely don't turn the page!

INTRODUCTION
The Unknown Blueprint of the Human Body

We are at an extraordinary juncture in human history where we are becoming ever more aware of critical aspects of our innate design. Insights from both the scientific and esoteric traditions are being confirmed regarding our physical reality that are, in a word, "astonishing." It's like we're awakening from a very long nap and slowly remembering who we really are!

For example, it has finally become widely accepted that what appears to be solidity of matter is actually mostly empty space (a whopping 99% in fact). Quantum physicists discovered that in the subatomic world, particles are not even predictably patterned constructs at all but waves of light energy of varying frequencies (this is what I refer to throughout this book as "light quotient.") Today, science recognizes that matter is light which only appears to be solid. This is radically different to what was commonly accepted just a few years ago.

Another mind-blowing realization comes from research into human DNA which reveals that what has been traditionally referred to as "junk DNA" is actually a very critical part of our genetic make-up that has merely been rendered "obsolete" by our lack of understanding and use.

The good news is that what these new findings (which are not "new" per se to the universe, just to _us_ as they have simply gone unrecognized until now) unmask is that we are powerful in ways we have only daydreamed about. Our full, original blueprint which we still carry, albeit in a dormant state (the part that has been labeled, "junk DNA"), contains codes that enable us to reawaken to a much richer potential.

Curiously, two of the most fundamental elements of our world – our human DNA blueprint and the building blocks of atoms – are radically different than what we thought they were just a few years ago. It is these findings about our sub-atomics and our DNA that, combined, become the guiding force of *The New Energy Body*.

These new understandings have changed everything, calling for nothing short of a complete re-evaluation of how we perceive ourselves, our world, our abilities and our future. This new perspective ripples through our relationship to the universe, how we treat, heal and feed our bodies and how we interface with all life on our planet.

What is The New Energy Body?

I call the state of being that we embody when we awaken the dormant DNA in our cells and raise the "light –quotient" of our sub-atomics "The New Energy Body." It literally draws a line in the sand between what we once perceived as our energy source and what we will now perceive as our energy source. We are at a crossroads – the opportunity to take the path of awakening the new energy body and leaving the old energy body – an outdated way of seeing, being and connecting behind. The *old* energy body is a body seeped in density, burdened by existence, relationships, fears and premature aging. The *New* Energy Body is a body that has been "enlightened" literally and figuratively.

There are 12 stages I have identified, which when used together, awaken The New Energy Body. I call them the "12 Sacred Stages" and you will be led through them stage-by-stage in Part II. Just as the old matter from food and environmental toxins can be cleared from our cells through our elimination channels, these steps can likewise cleanse the obstructions from our emotional and psychological lives that may be preventing us reaching our full potential.

As you will see, creating the New Energy Body is the ultimate detox process because it cleanses us of the density that prevents us from living in our wholeness – our whole joy, full energy and full power! When we are swimming in the toxicity of the modern lifestyle (negativity, fear and aggravation in addition to the obvious food wastes and pollution), we are an obstacle unto ourselves. We cannot see clearly enough to guide ourselves, much less lead others (including our children). Once the layers of density embedded in our physical cells and our emotional body are removed we can finally see our selves, our surroundings and our full potential clearly. It's like the light gets switched on in our proverbial "living room."

Those of you who have read my other books and are familiar with the dietary "transition" I advise might find it helps to apply this same approach to this process. It really should be approached as a transition too – in this case, transitioning from beings that struggle, get fat and age prematurely to beings filled with bliss who can finally have access to information that will liberate them to be masters of themselves and ultimately of whatever they wish to create.

In a very real way we go from being "merely human" and in some cases "sub-human" to "super-human." It's a simple case of evolution: we have suffered a mutation in our growth by these unprecedented modern factors and now we need to realign ourselves and correct the mutations so that we may flower into our full vitality and beauty.

Natalia Rose
June 12, 2007
New York City

PART I
The Principles of
The New Energy Body

"Those who are not shocked when they first come across quantum theory cannot possibly have understood it." – Niels Bohr

CHAPTER ONE
Principle #1: Get the Big Picture

There is so much that we cannot perceive from our 3-dimensional vantage point. Without full perception we cannot hope to accurately determine who we are, what we are or even where we are in the grand scope of things. We must realize as we stand today, we do not have the big picture.

One of the things that becomes abundantly obvious as we learn about the sub-atomics of matter is that just as matter is nothing more "concrete" than pulsating light-energy of various speeds, neither is the human body. Not only are our bodies not solid but we are also much more than the part of us that is materially manifested (i.e., seemingly solid, physical).

Modern man has long been limited by misconceptions about his world. The idea that we are more than material beings and that there is a governing force beyond us has always been relegated to religion. However more and more scientists are realizing that spirit is part of science – a key part if we are to accurately perceive our world. Albert Einstein once said, *"Even though the realms of religion and science in themselves are clearly marked off from each other, nevertheless here exist between the two strong reciprocal relationships and dependencies...The situation may be expressed by an image: Science without religion is lame, religion without science is blind."* It's ok to see ourselves as spiritual beings without associating it with any old energy religious undertone. Ancient civilizations were criticized for being superstitious because of their belief in spirit. Modern civilization is equally guilty of being superstitious of spirit by avoiding it out of fear of sounding religious or wacky. We are at the threshold of witnessing a new way to communicate about the spirit element of the human being that is educated, non threatening and non emotionally charged. How refreshing!

This part of us that remains unknown is potentially vast beyond our current conception. Therefore to hold fast to our static views despite the current findings does not make any common sense. What does make sense and what our generation is called to do with its vaster scope of knowledge is to expand beyond the static 3-Dimensional perspective and allow the next wave of perception to come through. We have to allow the bigger picture and let go of the more limited one. **The big picture is that we are limitless beings stuck in a limited perception**.

The Effect of Limited Perception: Suffering

Nearly all of our suffering is the cause of our birthright of limitless un-folding being stifled. We have been trained like monkeys to follow ideologies that have kept us under the thumb of all kinds of factions that would prefer to control us – in both subtle and obvious ways. I don't mean to imply that there is a giant conspiracy against human growth. I'm just pointing out that from our parents to our governments to the businesses that want us to buy their products, we are given lots of outside programming so we wind up acting in predictable ways which suits these factions even if it does not support our highest individual or communal good.

Just as the body sends out an alarm in the form of an ailment when it falls out of balance, we receive alarm signals in the form of suffering when our potential for growth either stalls or fails to take place because of factors we have accepted as our personal and communal limitations. In this way suffering can be seen and used as a guiding light for anything that is out of harmony in our lives. **If we pay attention to what our suffering is trying to tell us we can make the necessary corrections in our lives and bring an end to suffering.** But to do this we must expand our perspective to include the unseen realms along with what is more obviously right in front of us.

It has been suggested by yogis and metaphysicists for eons that we are not doomed to live and die in suffering and toil but that it's just our modern ways of living that have tricked us into following a distorted version of the truth. Our pain, anger and suffering come from this mass "illusion of limitation" which comes from being stuck in the 3rd dimension's perspective. I say "stuck" because we can have 3rd dimensional bodies and yet not be held down by the 3rd dimension if our perception of life is vaster than the 3rd dimension. We don't have to be stuck, you see. If you are presently stuck, recognize the bigger picture and know that you have created the glue holding yourself to that limited state of perception and you will eventually become unstuck.

While the modern material-focused cultures have continued on their wheel of suffering, many men and women have opted to awaken their light energy bodies and enjoy more divine states of being – some are rumored to have transmuted their bodies, ascended to higher realms or to have existed in states of constant nirvana.

To the average Western skeptic this is the stuff of stories. Its fun to imagine that there is an inner nectar to be enjoyed, but "it can't *really* be true," they conclude. So, the modern human carries on in fear and survival mode. Along the way, he goes deeper into his survival approach to life and becomes more distanced from the natural world. He takes in less fresh air, copious amounts of unnatural substances constantly (in the form of foods, drinks, pharmaceuticals, etc.), fills his mind with graphic images and his days with untold stresses. Relationships suffer, he loses touch with himself, and he dismisses his youthful caprices and loses more of his life force with every passing hour.

He completely misses out on the fun that being a human being is meant to be. He's like a battery powered toy that doesn't know he needs a battery and wonders why he is such a dud toy.

Meanwhile, it turns out not only are these accounts of a higher state of human existence true, they are within our reach. So what is it that these "immortals" know that we do not? Well, for one, they attribute their longevity to staying away from humans. This tongue-in-immortal-cheek rebuff actually reveals how much they know about the lost laws of science. They know the non-enlightened have a low light quotient that is in their best interest to avoid. They know that energetic fields resonate together. They realize that because of the laws of resonance which state that everything attunes to what is around it, they too would take on the offensive vibrational tone of modern humans. They keep away knowing that the energetic charges of the material, dense world are not favorable to sustaining the kind of vibe that correlates with immortality. You might say they keep their distance from the death imprint that modern man carries which could sully their life imprint. People have been snobby about lesser things.

But we don't have to move to the Himalayas or sell all our belongings and run around in magenta robes in order to reach the higher dimensional realms and become more conscious. We just have to "get the big picture" which is that we have been "in the dark" about things and we need to step into the light. We need to acknowledge that understanding only part of our world (having some light but not all light) is the key reason that we are so out of balance as individuals and as a global family.

The big picture is that we are powerful beyond anything we now commonly perceive and all the information is right under our noses – in fact it's even in the cells of our noses!

CHAPTER TWO
Principle #2: Plug Your DNA Cords Back In

It's officially true: one man's trash really is another man's treasure – at least where human DNA is concerned. Our DNA is comprised of 12 strands of protein fibers. Two of these 12 strands are recognized as having importance; the other ten strands were deemed useless simply because geneticists could not determine what they were for and to this day go by the term, "junk DNA." Unlike the two strands that were clearly linked to our physical genetic traits, when the ten additional strands failed to reveal their purpose, it was assumed they did not have one.

These orphaned DNA strands which, it turns out, are absolutely key to our full genetic understanding were carelessly dismissed and ignored. What would it mean to you to know that all that "junk DNA" is really a great power system that when working according to its original design tells a story of spinning rainbow Light that holds within it our coding for greater human power, our connection to our true home and the proof of realms far beyond the 3-dimensional world within which we perceive ourselves to be confined?   It's all there in a resplendent spiral pattern that we, in a world preoccupied with what we can make sense of physically, simply haven't understood!

It made such obvious common intellectual and instinctual sense to me that the 10 strands of DNA labeled "junk DNA" could not possibly really be junk! Like everything else in the body, nothing is dispensable or "extra." Everything plays an important role in ensuring that our physicality runs smoothly.

What I learned is that the two strands that we herald as our genetic blueprint only tell us about our physical imprint. **BUT, the other ten strands give us the rest of the picture of who we are!** Each of these strands corresponds to a different level of awareness – and thus a different dimension (if you like, dimensions can be thought of as different levels of awareness). This is critical to understanding the big picture of higher dimensions so let's look at it:

Imagine if you only knew the "up/down" dimension: your awareness would be stuck in that limited state of comprehending your world. From this limited perspective you couldn't possibly hope to know much about the world beyond. From the vantage point of 3-D awareness, we see out and in, up and down and left to right but that's not all that's out there!

By awakening the other ten strands of our DNA we have the opportunity to then connect with the other dimensions and know ourselves and our world more fully. It's like what would happen if "up/down" folks were suddenly made aware of "in/out" and "left/right." They would know their world more completely.

I'm not trashy; you're not trashy!

DNA conducts light through its structure and stores this information in its double helix "ladder" design. The light of our genetic coding holds the patterning for our **physical** structure. But this is only part of what we know of our DNA – less than 10%. The other 90%+ of our DNA has been labeled, "junk."

So what does this other 90% of superconductor, intelligence contain as it sits there in the dust-bin of the halls of science and human consciousness? Seems it contains something rather unworthy of the junk pile. Its coding tells a magical story of who we really are and the unlimited abilities that have gone overlooked along our would-be information highways. Fortunately, it's not too late to switch the power button back on and plug all that rejected DNA back into its rightful sockets to revive us so we can finally tap the truth of our nature and abilities.

By now I'm sure you're curious to know what the other ten strands (five double helixes) that have been junked represent. The best explanation comes from a source called Integrated Energy Therapy. Because they have phrased it so well, I am going to quote directly from them.[1]

"**The 2nd Pair:** governs our emotional body. It controls our genetic emotional profile as well as our predisposition to certain emotional conditions. For example, it governs our EQ (our emotional intelligence quotient), determines whether we will be a type A or a type B personality and determines whether we will be introverted or extroverted.

"**The 3rd Pair DNA:** governs our mental body. It controls our genetic mental profile and determines whether our mental energy be directed toward logical, linear, rational thinking (as in a scientist or an engineer) or toward the intuitive, artistic expression. Furthermore, it controls whether we will be primarily optimistic or primarily pessimistic.

"**The 4th Pair DNA:** governs our soul. It controls our karmic patterning and our genetic soul profile. (Karmic patterning refers to the karmic pre-conditioning that we have brought into this lifetime to work with and master. Specifically, it includes karmic wounds, issues or lessons that were not resolved or completed in past lifetime experiences and which will re-manifest in this lifetime to give us with an opportunity to resolve them). Genetic soul profile governs our soul's mission. It determines what soul level archetypal pattern we will have. For example will we be destined to be a leader, healer, builder, teacher, student, warrior, monastic, parent, etc? Furthermore, it contains a profile of the

---

[1] Integrated Energy Therapy: http://www.integratedenergytherapy.net/12_strand_dna2.asp

experiences we are to have, the wisdom we are to develop, the spiritual strengths we are to master, the service we are to provide to others and the path we are to take to find pure joy).

"**The 5th Pair DNA**: governs our soul cluster and controls the movement and timing of specific souls within a soul cluster to seek and find each other to the mutual fulfillment of their soul's purpose.

"**The 6th Pair DNA:** governs all of creation and aligns your 12-strand DNA with divine will."

Modern science acknowledges that we live in a world of three dimensions of space plus one dimension of time (known as the 4th dimension). This concept has defined everything we understand about our world. It is however, a limited perspective because there are more dimensions than these four and they are around us and within us at this very moment.

Thankfully, there have been scientist and metaphysicists who have not accepted this limited construct as their exclusive definition of our world; they suggest that the existing dimensions are probably no fewer than 11 and potentially infinite in number. [2]

---

[2] Physics' String theory shows us that Space is dynamic and changeable; it challenges everything we know about our world, revealing that extra dimensions, rips in the fabric of space, and parallel universes actually exist. I recommend watching the PBS/Nova videos on String Theory: http://www.pbs.org/wgbh/nova/elegant/media2/3014_q_01.html

With each dimensional step up, we likewise move "up" toward more refined, brilliant light because we transcend the density of the 3-D experience. As we achieve these rarified states, our cells literally oscillate more rapidly and become more radiantly light containing. We move through the electromagnetic light spectrum away from the slower frequency longer light waves into the invisible faster frequency shorter, light waves.

A thought to ponder: perhaps what we refer to as going "up to heaven" was not intended to meant going "up" in the sky per se but rather "up" dimensionally speaking which is also "up" on the vibrational scale which holds more light and thus more information which makes us feel more "uplifted" because with each higher vibe and dimension there is more bliss. So this "up" idea has to do with dimensions and vibrations (not just altitude).

Let's take a look at the known and the lesser known but intuited dimensions which correspond with the 12 strands of DNA:

The Known Dimensions:

The 1st **Dimension** is that of the earth and the mineral kingdom. This can be correlated (as above so below) to the bone and teeth system in the human body. Spatially, this is the "up/down."

The 2nd **Dimension** is that of the plant kingdom which connects with our nervous system (communication network). Spatially, this is left/right."

The 3rd **Dimension** is that of man's consciousness. Spatially, this is "in/out."

The 4th Dimension is that of time and thought-astral expression. Science refers to this as the dimension of TIME. Just like the 3rd dimension controls the 2^{nd,} the 4th dimension has "dominion" over the 3rd. In this way it is the field around the 3rd dimensional plane that governs it.

The Intuited Dimensions

The 5th Dimension is that of awareness of soul and spirit.

The 6th Dimension is that of the morphogenic field – where thought, color and sound take on geometric shapes.

The 7th Dimension is that of group consciousness or ONENESS. It is also known as the dimension of sound harmonics.

The 8th dimension is that of infinity – it is where the void can be experienced merging with creative power. There is complete unity of all things. It is the figure eight – the symbol and experience of infinity.

The 9th Dimension is as far as conscious can go before merging with the fullness of our Source light. This is where we begin to lose our sense of individuality (only to gain a much greater awareness of our self if we hang in there and continue).

The 10th Dimension is the experience of merging individual consciousness with All That Is. We feel ourselves blending into the Source.

The 11th Dimension is direct connection to Source. We are at the final stage of merging before we are fully conscious in …

The 12th Dimension where we fully perceive ourselves again as SOURCE. Here we find ourselves in full "God-head" consciousness.

So, what we have here is a concept that we are actually connected to many dimensions that we are not aware of. Further, as we grow in awareness of them and reactivate our DNA which has a strand connected to each one of these dimensions, we will then have access to these dimensions which we can experience as we unfold into this grander concept of ourselves.

On one hand this may come off as a spiritual theory. But this is where science and spirituality ultimately cross paths. Science explains our world and if our world leads us to plausible theories that seem somehow spiritual at their essence this does not make the theories any less scientific. If our world is proven to be mechanical and random at the end of our seeking then spirituality will have to concede thus; if, on the other hand the spiritual intelligence is indeed creating our world, it will be the role of science to validate that discovery.

Plugging in these additional ten strands of DNA can be triggered in a number of ways that are all fun, expansive, pleasurable and fulfilling as we will discuss in the next section. If you like you can try the following exercise to start expanding your awareness and your limitations:

Exercise for inter-dimensional perception: Close your eyes and perceive your surroundings. Now, bit by bit carry your perception outward (spherically all around you) such that you are perceiving and acknowledging your connection with the vastness of the universe. Perceive beyond our solar system in all directions. Perhaps you will perceive other solar systems, galaxies. Move out and out with your perception and feel the physical and mental experience of perceptual exploration. The more you do this, the more you will realize your place in this vastness, the sense of you being a part of it all and able to access it all at will. When you move into stages of connecting with greater vastness, you are stimulating your dormant DNA strands that correspond with that dimension to reconnect. You are entering that dimension with the sheer power of your awareness. Feel you mind open and your cells fill with the bliss of this vast expansion. If you feel fear, allow that too. But know that love is all there is and all that's real and you are completely supported and safe.

CHAPTER THREE
Principle #3: Light Takes Shape

"All of creation is moving Light. Sacred Geometry is the blueprint of Creation and the genesis of all form. It is an ancient science that explores and explains the energy patterns that create and unify all things and reveals the precise way that the energy of Creation organizes itself. On every scale, every natural pattern of growth or movement conforms inevitably to one or more geometric shapes.

As you enter the world of Sacred Geometry you begin to see as never before the wonderfully patterned beauty of Creation. The molecules of our DNA, the cornea of our eye, snow flakes, pine cones, flower petals, diamond crystals, the branching of trees, a nautilus shell, the star we spin around, the galaxy we spiral within, the air we breathe, and all life forms as we know them emerge out of timeless geometric codes. Viewing and contemplating these codes allow us to gaze directly at the lines on the face of deep wisdom and offers up a glimpse into the inner workings of the Universal Mind and the Universe itself." – Oliver Markley

All light contains the blueprint for expression. In the realms between source and physicality are etheric expressions of light known as sacred geometry. Sacred geometry is shapes and their underlying mathematics that reflect the divine characteristics – they are the patterns that hold the information for the thing the intelligence wants to express/create. This is why we call them "sacred" – they carry the divine imprint and blueprint. Remember that shapes are ruled by the 6th Dimension, the morphogenic field where thought, color and sound take on geometric shapes!

But to put it more simply, when you look at the shape of things in nature, they are all governed by the intelligence supporting them which carries the intention for their form into physicality. Even though everything in nature looks very unique, the underlying patterns that created them (the codings that carry out their form every season when they bloom) have a whole lot in common. I like to think of this signature that is all over the natural world as the "fingerprint" of the original light/intelligence: the "Source Light."

You see, as it turns out, what we perceive in every structure in the natural world reveals geometries upon geometries. Light creates forms that are either circular, spiral or linear but they all follow the same fundamental mathematics.

This mathematical core is called the Fibonacci Sequence[3] and within this geometric explanation is the underlying code of all of life.[4] Within it we find the blueprints for the nautilus shell, rams horns, our fingerprints, our DNA and even our very Milky Way galaxy! Geometries upon geometries, as above so below, worlds upon worlds…

Geometries upon Geometries

The geometries are the structures that hold light instructions and coding (the blueprint) to direct the desired material thing's materialization. This is how divine thought becomes manifested into 3-D form. Each thought becomes encoded with an etheric blueprint which unfolds in this dimension and we perceive it to be real. This is why it is so important to understand the mystical truths of our world. If we miss this key law we wind up creating unconsciously – not realizing that it is our thoughts, our intentions that spring from our beliefs that are giving form to our reality and are the cause of our effect, the seeds of our experiences.

We'll discuss more about how creation actually takes place in the next chapter, **but understanding the geometries that govern shape of things in our world is**

---

[3] 0, 1, 1, 2, 3, 5, 8, 13, 21, 34, 55, 89, 144, 233, 377, 610, 987, 1597, 2584, 4181, 6765, 10946, 17711, 28657, 46368, 75025… Note: sometimes this sequence is considered to start at $F_1 = 1$, but it is more common to include $F_0 = 0$.

4 If you divide a straight line so that about 61% of it is on one side and 39% on the other, you will find that the ration of the large portion to the small is the same as the ratio of the overall line to the large portion. Rectangles made with these proportions can be subdivided endlessly. This self-mirroring proportion was essential to the art and architecture of the Greeks; it is very pleasing to the mind's eye and was used extensively, including in the design of the Parthenon. http://fusionanomaly.net/goldenmean.html

essential to fully grasping creation because it ties the pillars of creation (sound, vibration, light and shape) together. The geometric design is the expression in shape form of a given thought/energy vibration just as words are the audible expression of the sounds formed by a given energetic thought pattern. In fact, to go a step further, the written word (letters) hold the physical blueprint of the sound pattern that the specific thought-vibration makes! Everything that we see materially has a geometric, etheric underlying blueprint.

In terms of your physicality, the geometries express the vibrational form that is you – right down to the perfectly self-replicating DNA. This is why I am going to such lengths to emphasize the sacred geometries at play in our world and how they originate in a non-material place – in the etheric blueprint before they become form.

All form starts out as a thought vibe which contains sound which contains shapes which create form. There is a definite ladder that leads down to what we experience as form and which can take us right back up to where all form originated.

Our human shape is encased in the larger geometric patterns as illustrated in Leonardo Di Vinci's Vitruvian Man. Yet we can step into smaller and smaller encasement patterns as we go deeper into the body. As with everything in the universe, there is a macrocosmic and a microcosmic perspective within all things. For example, there is the body as a whole (macrocosmic), the organs taken separately (microcosmic) -- within that encasement are crystalline bone structures, cells within bones and, the ultimate geometric pattern: the double helix within the cell which carries our physio-spiritual genetic coding (the ultra microcosmic level as it relates to our body) – yet they all follow the same geometric laws.

There is structure at the most minute levels of creation – for example every drop of water holds a crystallized structure. Imagine: every cell in our body is shaped by a thought from somewhere, although it may be a dimension unseen by our present faculties!

In *The Biology of Belief*, Bruce Lipton writes, "Are the repetitive images observed in Nature simply coincidence? I believe the answer is, 'no.' He goes on to explain his view on a geometric concept termed a "fractal," defined as irregular and fragmented self similar shapes in a paper entitled, Fractal Evolution.[5] "In Nature," he writes, "most inorganic and organic structures express an 'irregular' pattern. However, within the apparent chaos of the irregularities, one finds that the irregular structures are 'regularly' repeated (i.e., they show a form of order). For example, the pattern of branching in a tree's twig is often the same pattern of branching that is observed on the tree's trunk. The pattern of branching of a major river is identical to the pattern of branching observed along its smaller tributaries. The pattern of branches along the bronchus is a reiteration of the pattern of airway branches along the smallest bronchioles. Similar images of reiterated branching patterns in the body are

---

[5] http://www.brucelipton.com/article/fractal-evolution

revealed in the arterial and venous blood vessels and peripheral nervous system...A structural characteristic of fractals is relatively simple to understand: fractals exhibit a reiterated pattern of 'structures' nested within one another. Each smaller structure is a miniature, but not necessarily an exact version of the larger form. Fractal mathematics emphasizes the relation between the patterns seen in the whole and the patterns seen in parts of that whole. For example, the pattern of twigs on a branch resembles the pattern of limbs branching off of the trunk. Fractal objects can be represented by a 'box' within a 'box,' within a 'box,' within a 'box,' etc. If one knows the parameters of the first 'box,' then one is automatically provided with the basic pattern that characterizes all of the other (larger or smaller) 'boxes.' Humans are a fractal image of society, cells are a fractal image of the human. In fact, cells are a fractal image of society as well."

With so many competing thoughts moving around in our heads all day and their intentions which are sent out on subconscious, conscious and super-conscious levels at once, there is a lot that gets created at all levels of our experience from our individual consciousness to that of others and ultimately as materialized by what is called our "group consciousness." This is what creates form and experiences from cultures to nations from modes of fashion to whether there will be war or peace.

Some of what is created gets its blueprint from a source rooted in wholeness and peace which will surely embody wholeness and peace in its materialization. But some of what is created will come from pain, anger and fear which will have an altogether different structure. We see this type of energy take shape in atrophied geometries: from the formation of a __cancer cell__ to the chaotic energies building around an angry exchange between people or countries to the very breakdown in our natural world that is manifested in mutated living things. We even see it manifested as clutter if we have cluttered lives.

We cannot separate thought from matter – our thought projections from our physical state of being. Our cosmic consciousness projects our global state of being. Sacred geometries must be understood in order to understand the thought behind the materialization of all we experience. The shape that things take always mirrors the thoughts from which they originate (the origin of a thought is belief)!

The Original Form of Sacred Geometry: The Torus

Have you ever noticed that all fruit is generally round or cylindrical in shape with a lifeline running through its inner core? The core of the fruit is the lifeline of the fruit. Look at everything from an orange to a pineapple, a grape, kiwi, cherry, nectarine, even a banana -- they all share this structural dynamic.

A fruit's inner lifeline is a clearly imprinted, delineating passage way that runs vertically along the length of the fruit. The top of the fruit is typically masculine – think of the phallic design of the apple stem or pineapple top. This is a connection to the vine of course but we'll look at that later. The bottom is receptive and feminine (either flat or concave). Remind you of a battery perhaps? There is the positive (masculine) end and the negative (feminine) end.

Through this core, energy enters into the top of the plant (the stem/vine/etc) and pours its energy through the fruit. The female charge (-) feeds into the masculine charge (+) which together comprise the vine and the root structure which represent the conception and birthing power in all life as the male and female energies coming together in co-creation. Meanwhile, sunlight (which is a masculine energy) brings Life Force Energy to the fruit from the outside through the receptive end of the fruit and the skin (which is also feminine in nature) as well as through the receptive earth (the famously feminine, "mother earth"). Therefore, the fruit perfectly illustrates the primal pattern of energy that runs up and down the fruit in a circular route constantly feeding and receiving energy. This pattern of energy becomes the shape of the fruit to reveal the original shape of life. This primal and key pattern is the "Torus."

The fruit itself takes on this torus shape – it is the solid embodiment of the energetic cycle in the ethers. It is the perfect example of light taking shape – first on the etheric plane from the patterns of the energy flow and then physically in the solidity that comes from that flow from pole to pole.

The torus pattern of energy is the electromagnetic design of every living thing. The mammalian spinal column, vine, stalk and trunk of the plant is the pathway where the Life Force Energy of the male and the zero point energy of the female meet to generate life. The male energy flows from the crown to the root and spherically out and around and the female energy flows spherically out and up through the root toward the crown and around again. You might say that sexual energy is all around us!

The human design is also structured around this great column of energy that runs down the spinal column while simultaneously up the spinal column. Imagine that, following the image of the Torus when the energy hits the bottom of the column it splits in two and re-circulates dually at opposite sides of the body. The same happens with the energy entering from the bottom going up. So you have this donut-like flow-pattern all around the body.

Where does the energy that feeds both the top and bottom of the spinal column come from? The one that feeds into the top of the spinal column comes through the brain from the crown of the head and carries the electromagnetic current (Life Force Energy) from the higher realms from all the way back "up" the scales of frequency to the Source of all life. (a.k.a. "God the Father.") This is considered a masculine energy. The energy that feeds into the base of the spine comes from the earth energies is considered to embody the feminine energy – thus, the "Goddess" the "Earth Mother," the "Great Nurturer." It's a constant dance of attraction between the male and female energy poles. You might say it's the ultimate pole dance!

The receptivity of this power that we are designed to be fed by is based on the individual. In my previous book, *Raw Food Life Force Energy*, I explained that the state of the physical body is a reflection of how your energy body is flowing and vise versa. Let's now take that concept a step further to reveal that the energy potential that will be manifested by the individual is dependent upon his or her openness and awareness of their potential. Lack of awareness itself can diminish the flow just like the lack of awareness of proper breathing hampers the intake of oxygen. What wonders a little awareness of where your energy is coming from can do!

Imagine for a moment being fed Life Force Energy through the top of your head and through your root and vice versa and your whole being will begin to awaken, pulsating to this sensation as you literally bring more life force into the body. Note that it's the earth and the seed (the feminine and the masculine together) that create life. This aspect of creation can be seen in all things and when you awaken this in the body and in your perception of your own capacity to create. Prepare to be amazed by what you discover!

Are the geometries of DNA meaningful in any of this? You bet! The geometries behind the double helix are loaded with clues to our origins! We've established that geometric structures hold the form of the blueprint for materialization into 3-D form. Well, the ultimate coding for Light's blueprint is human DNA – it is the most advanced blueprint in 3-D form.

DNA holds crystallized living shapes created by information patterns. These structures which are simply light-information patterns in physical form can be seen in every part of our being from the liquid crystalline structures of the water in our body to the "solid" crystallized geometric forms called minerals which make up our bones. This "Light Information" has a communication network whose Head Quarters can be found in every cell. It's our physical blueprint for Light's desired expression within us, our DNA. It also follows the spiral sequencing of the Fibonacci/Phi pattern!

This is all to say that the thing that determines our geometries, our cells, tissues, organs and other structures as well as our behavior and health destiny is in itself a geometric coding.   However, this geometric coding holds keys that empower us to adjust the coding through the strands that are connected to our mind, emotions and divine realms, which is why I prefer to call it our "physio-spiritual" genetic coding. This implies the unity of our physicality and our spirituality.

Each step on the ladder up the sacred geometries of the DNA spiral reveal all the steps we took to land ourselves in physical form as well as those steps we can take to get ourselves back up the ladder to our true origin when we are done exploring physical form. Each cell holds a 12-strand DNA matrix in a spiraling ladder design, which indicates that each cell has the potential to express all 12 steps and strands of the DNA matrix. In this way, each cell has a potential destiny that is greater than what it reaches on its own. It's the cosmic code: as above so below; as below so above.

The Shape of Sound-Vibration

Everything in existence has a corresponding sound. Every sound has a corresponding shape. Every shape carries Light in varying intensities. You are a sound that has become a shape that carries Light. Seen the other way, you are Light which as been down-stepped into geometric patterns which spell out vibratory rhythms that can be seen as matter by the human eye.

Your personal sound/light holds the architectural design of the present state of your *current* physical body. Before clearing myself of a good deal of inharmonious vibrations, I was plagued with jumbling my speech when I was nervous or what I now call being "out of tune." It was embarrassing - my speech would run off out of control – it ran ahead of me on an uncontrollable trajectory!

My voice, the tenor, power, frequency changed significantly once I became grounded in my New Energy Body. Not only did I stop slurring and stumbling my speech, but I took on the tonality that expressed itself in speech with a measured cadence that reflected my new, improved inner cadence. This was pretty remarkable to me because it proved that the sound that comes out of the human being (be it harmonious or disparate) was directly reflecting my discordant inner being "sounding off."   In my case the sound-vibrations my geometric patterns were giving off proved how maladroit the geometric patterns of my physical being were back then. I have a much clearer, more melodious voice now reflecting my improved geometric blueprint. However, I can always tell if I am falling out of balance or vibrationally compromised because my vocal expression will start to suffer. This is the concept behind vocally attuning to the OHM sound. When we make this sound we can take an instant read on our inner-harmony telling us how in or out of tune we are and so we can make the necessary adjustments. Think about how a child's voice changes in tenor and tone as it grows into its adult geometric light body. Its new architecture makes a new sound!

In this way you can see how your light and geometric blueprint determine your physical shape. If you do not like the shape of the light you're reflecting, you can make improvements to it by simply raising your Light Quotient (your LQ) through several avenues: 1) a more Light-filled diet; 2) a kinder, more loving approach to life; and 3) surrounding yourself with a more Light and Life Force Energy-rich environment (local, relationships, job, home); and 4) Conscious, specific Light-raising thoughts and meditations (see stages 2 and 6).

Increase the Light in your soul, physicality and environment and your shape will respond because at the risk of sounding pedantic, Light Takes Shape! The implications here are multifold and certainly include our own ability to create the shape of our cells (healthy as opposed to distrophied or cancerous) as well as our whole body!

From a microcosmic perspective, the structure of every cell in your body is patterned by the Light quotient it carries. From a macrocosmic perspective, your whole body's shape and abilities are determined by the Light quotient it carries. Increase the Light quotient and every cell will step into line with that increase – improving the size, structure and radiance of your skin, girth and organs. Our earth, solar system and universe are all likewise affected by the amount of pure, Life Force Energy it has in its realm. It can be more blissful and light-filled, or darker, denser and sadder.

This tells us something pretty remarkable – we can change our bodies, inside and out, cell by cell, organ by organ based on nothing more than the "resonance" of the energy we carry. We can bring a more bliss-filled Light-sound-geometric force into the body that can transform us into what we most desire. If we want to move into states of being that are more beautiful, joyful and radiantly healthy, we need simply tune into a frequency that brings this quality of Light to us. We do this through our physical, mental and emotional faculties. When all of these faculties tune in to the frequency we desire, our whole being shifts into this transformed state and voila we are that much better off. Think of it as sacred physio-spiritual surgery!

Light magnitude + Thought intention = Geometric expression = Physical Crystalline Structure

In his book, Messages from Water, Dr. Masaru Emoto discovered that by placing certain messages on bottles of water, the crystalline structure of the water changed to reflect a geometric pattern reflective of the energy the word or phrase carried. We can deduce from this that water is a mirror-image conduit of thought-energy. This means that if we are made up of mostly water, we too will physically mirror the thought structures and environment we place ourselves within. Light in this case becomes manifested through thought that is physically rendered through the crystalline geometric patterns which vibrate at the intensity of the light it carries mixed with the intention of the thought.

Anger, hate and misery dystrophy the integrity of our crystalline shapes damaging the crystalline foundations that make up the majority of the body – namely the bones and water. Imagine the healing we could generate in the super-swift conductivity of water throughout our bodies if we consistently embody thoughts of love, beauty and joy.   How the crystalline geometric patterns reflected would captivate with their symmetry, harmony and dazzlingly treasured geometric structures!

A body made up of perfected, high integrity geometries comes from self love and will inevitably glow inside and out. The opposite is also true. This tells us that love and beauty really do come from within. We love ourselves into beauty.

How misguided that in today's world we do the opposite? We sooner hate ourselves into beauty salons and diet centers only to continuously look even more weathered, burdened and maligned (though we find endless ways to avoid being honest with ourselves about this pattern generation after generation.) The torment goes on as the answers seem to be beyond us and old age with its mounting burdens and discomforts takes over.   This, my friends, is not how it has to be. A candid peek into the blueprint of the intended energy body offers very real solutions to the illusions we have endured that have made us feel ugly, lethargic and heavy.

What I am here to tell you is that you can heal yourself. You can be more beautiful. You can unlock doors to radiance and leave behind the old mentality of need for expensive creams, brutal exercise, diet regimes and painful self-hatred. Create the body of your dreams by loving it into existence – literally.

You are your own Alchemist: You can take your heavy body of "lead" and transform it into a vehicle of pure etheric golden light. All you need is the Philosopher's stone which is the pure vibration of love that you are (but may have temporarily forgotten). Some of you will want to further explore the science and mathematics behind sacred geometries to help you accept this concept intellectually (this is the male path of the intellect.) Others will immediately *feel* the transformation in their bodies when they start to increase the energy of love beginning in the heart move through the body. (this is the path of feminine intuition.)

We will soon go into detail about shifting the frequency of your physical and emotional being. All the while, keep in mind that in order for your body and life to be different they need to broadcast the frequency of the frequency it wants to bring into it so this change can take place. You cannot broadcast the frequency of hate, fear and a bad case of the "uglies" and expect to hone into the frequency of love, security and beauty.

"Your beliefs become your thoughts
Your thoughts become your words
Your words become your actions
Your actions become your habits
Your habits become your values
Your values become your destiny"
- Mahatma Gandhi

CHAPTER FOUR
Principle #4: The New Energy Body Can Create!

ALL THAT IS is ours to create with once we are unified with our highest consciousness.

All around us is energy. The very sea of air we swim in is a realm of pure energy. Energy in and of itself is not positive or negative. It is neutral. It is, like molding clay or a paint brush and canvass, for us to take and design into whatever we fancy seeing, being or experiencing!

There are two creative laws of the universe that will help us understand how it is that we create.

The first is the law of affinity (like attracts like). The other is that opposites attract. It would seem that these two laws would most certainly contradict each other. But actually they work together. Let me explain:

Universal manifestation Law #1

Where light is concerned same poles attract: This is the concept, "*like attracts like.*" Behind the actual vibratory light energy that creates and carries the vibratory blueprint (the egg) lies a thought or feeling that attracts that vibratory energy (the blueprint.) This feeling or thought originates from a **belief**. In this way, we should recognize our beliefs as being the originators of our creations. Instead of trying to falsely attempt to mold our thoughts and feelings, we are much better served by changing our beliefs so that our beliefs are good breeders for attracting "like" vibrational energies.

Universal manifestation Law #2

Where light and matter are concerned, opposite poles attract. This is the concept, "*opposites attract.*" Once the vibratory note is sounded (the vibratory note is feminine) the law of attraction comes into play because atoms (which are masculine by their magnetic nature) are then drawn to the vibratory note (which is feminine in nature) and have their structure dictated via the geometric blueprint held by the geometric light pattern within the energetic vibration that is broadcast from the thought/feeling from the mind in which it originates (the creator.) Thus the atoms are attracted (opposites-male/female-attract) to the vibratory light blueprint and take their destined shape. You might think of the light-vibration blueprint as the egg "holding" the substance for hatching in the material realm. It's all very magical – yet we do it every moment.

"Let us guard our thoughts for from them our future is born." - Almine Barton

<u>So let's get this manifestation thing straight:</u> Beliefs create emotions and thoughts which create feelings that carry a vibration which attract the blueprint facsimile of that vibration/thought/feeling. The blueprint of that feeling (held together by its specific geometric structure) attracts atoms which, when bonded together in this cosmic magnetism, take form. This is the cycle. Now that you know it and understand it you can see it at work in your life and make it work for you! Have fun!!

Notice that in the above quote from Mahatma Gandhi *he did not say your thoughts become your beliefs. It's always the other way around* – YOUR BELIEFS CREATE YOUR THOUGHTS. Gandhi was absolutely correct. As much as we try the mold our experience by directing our thoughts, unless our beliefs are in sync with that thought our life experiences will continue to match the beliefs we do hold. Our beliefs have to be changed for our experience to change because our belief shapes our thoughts which become the blueprint that attracts the form of our experience. A thought might ignite a new belief but it will not supplant old beliefs which are the determining factor. Beliefs come from what we hold in our knowingness – our DNA connections with our emotional body, memories and inherited beliefs encoded in the DNA

With so much talk about creating one's own reality and the power of thought at from popular movies and books like "The Secret" the laws of manifestation run the risk of getting a bit of the "common touch" as it were. There is more to it than simply feeling and imagining what you want. To suggest this is all there is to it would be offering up false hope (to my mind there is nothing worse than false hope). Like a raw food diet, creation must be done properly with the utmost attention to personal impeccability for it to be rewarding. For this reason I would like to highlight a few basic keys that will ensure you know how to use this knowledge in its highest design:

1) All thought and feeling come first from BELIEF. You can try to bend your mind to envision your dreams and affirm things to your conscious mind but UNLESS YOU HAVE "DETOXIFIED" THE UNDERLYING PROGRAMMING you'll continue to have the same set of circumstances because you will still be broadcasting the same old messages which attract the same old stories to your life. The only way to be sure your beliefs are sound is to "cancel" and "burn" these programs per the exercises on pg. 106.

2) Forcing "positive thinking" is counter intuitive because it represses your real thoughts and feelings which both magnify the negative thought giving those negative thoughts more power and repressing them inside the individual making the pain deeper and more acute. I cannot stress enough how important it is to ALLOW our natural thoughts and feelings because when we do this we can shine the light on them, find

Bruce Lipton writes in The Biology of Belief (Mountain of Love/Elite Books; pg 169),

> *The conscious mind is the "self," the voice of our own thoughts. It can have great visions and plans for a future filled with love, health, happiness and prosperity. While we focus our consciousness on happy thoughts, who is running the show? The subconscious. How is the subconscious going to manage our affairs? Precisely the way it was programmed. The subconscious mind's behaviors when we are not paying attention may not be of our own creation because most of our fundamental behaviors were downloaded without question from observing other people. Because subconscious-generated behaviors are not generally observed by the conscious mind, many people are stunned to hear that they are "just like their mom or their dad," the people who programmed their subconscious minds.*

3) Be wary of the material focus: many of the messages coming from today's "creation enthusiasts" simply reinforce materialism, vanity,

competition and power. You see, we need to stop feeding the programming that money or a romantic relationship will bring us the satisfaction we seek. They never do. We must stop seeking to fulfill ourselves from the outside. So you manifest money – a lot of money, a gorgeous spouse, a new career or position in power – so what? Do you think you are going to have any more peace than you have today? It may thrill you initially but what when you come down off that high? You might manage to get what you want, but like a kid on Christmas, after a short while you have to bring your toy into the real world and live with yourself and your inner chatter again.

You cannot be truly happy until you are at peace with everything around you. This comes not from visualizing and manifesting material wealth, power or recognition but from removing the old programs that have you imprisoned in a perception of life where material wealth is the goal. The irony is that when you experience this there are no needs, no desires. You have more than the sum of all your desires.

When you can manifest a reality that has no visceral response to outside fulfillment (positive or negative) you are on the right track. When you are free of the sway of other people's ideas and in your full essence then you will experience real power that cannot be taken from you. You will live without fear, without limits, without judgments and criticisms, without other people's projections and ideologies. This may seem impossible to you now and it is not required that you be pure of thought and desire and completely unaffected by others in the early stages. That will come with practice and focused intent. I only say this to point out the difference between real power and the illusion of power and to emphasize that using the tools of manifestation to create wealth for the sake of wealth is never going to slay your inner dragons.

4) Finally, if we are focused on abundance for the sake of personal wealth and power we continue on that unfathomably misguided trajectory that has taken us away from our unity as a planet. It's the "ME ME ME" attitude that created so much separation and has made our lives so empty and distant to begin with. To focus on manifesting for the sake of more material comforts we will continue to distance ourselves from each other – deepening the wound that has already been made among mankind, races and governments. When we manifest from the perspective of "what serves me serves all and what serves all will serve me" we will start to heal ourselves and reunify communally, leading to even greater ecstatic joy.

So what stands in our way of this ultimate co-creatorship? Just our beliefs. We don't like to think of ourselves as puppets that do as we are told and who are managed and directed, yet if we recognize that everything we do is part of pre-designed framework of belief structures that did not originate with us but that we simply accepted for various reasons, we must acknowledge that we tend toward robotic or puppet like behavior. It's time to cut the strings and the wires and step into our full self-sovereignty.

We can still create a beautiful life for ourselves, including a beautiful place to live and lots of wonderful people to share it with but it needs to come from a different place within us – not from our pain, our sense of lack or not being good enough – but from a grounded, deeply connected, heart-centered place. For this reason, I suggest holding off on actively creating until you've mastered the previous stages and cleansed the muck out of your beliefs that might undermine your creative efforts.

CHAPTER FIVE
Principle #5: The Golden Key

"Heart-based feelings and emotions inside our bodies changes the DNA inside our bodies producing quantum effects in the field beyond our body that change our physical world"-- Gregg Braden[6]

The reason physically transforming my cells and experiencing this literal high was so meaningful to activating my DNA is because when one moves into higher states of being, one naturally releases anger and fears which are the two big strong holds that our social programming has on us, limiting us. <u>When this happens, we can open to our true essence. This "essence" is the golden key to</u>

---

[6] *The God Code, The Quantum Hologram CD*

all that we are.   This is critical to receiving the golden key to full DNA activation and what you will learn about in this chapter.

By feeling better about my body and experiencing so much energy my world brightened. This led to me identifying less with the anger and fear that came with the self criticism, discomforts and insecurities of my life experience prior to my physical cleansing back when I was so far removed from my pure essence and seeped in my programmed beliefs.

By removing the programming we become our authentic vibration – our **pure essence** comes through. We are all unique but at our authentic, pure essence we are all made of exactly the same thing: pure love. When I speak of pure love, I am not talking about a concept or an abstract emotion. I am talking about a very real substance --- a vibratory material which may not be visible in the visible light spectrum but is nevertheless real.

When you fully grasp the concept that we are mostly space (99% space) and that the rest of us (all that is real – though ironically unseen) is vibratory energy you can understand why this personal "essence" is so challenging to define using the English vocabulary without invoking religious undertones or poetic expression.

This essence though, when you start to tap it (and you will if you just give it a chance to awaken through the stages in the next section) is what will finally open up your whole world and transform you into the most powerful, beautiful, joyful person you can be. It awakens our dormant DNA strands because it is the full expression of ourselves which resonates with the complete DNA structure we are so gifted to have been created with. It makes "switching ourselves back on" automatic! **When you can start to feel and embody your own essence anything dormant that resonates with that essence will awaken** (including sunnier parts of your personality, latent talents and even the youthful look and feeling that you put to pasture when you were put to pasture)!

This is the most real, authentic part of us; it is the part of us that presents us with the greatest opportunities for growth and expanded perception. Therefore, by removing the rubbish that you previously (unconsciously) identified with and stepping more fully into the pure love that we are, we awaken all levels of our DNA, create beautiful lives of unselfish abundance that reflect that love (the laws of resonance and attraction), and ultimately, we exist fully in the sweet nectar of our own precious essence.

Love can then be understood, not just as an emotion, a desire or an expectation of another but as the most refined level of vibratory energy in existence. So, if at our essence, we carry the essence of our creator, we can focus on that essence and power instead of old beliefs, labels and conditioning and watch the miracles in our life start to replace the suffering and pain. Love essence refines your Light Quotient which triggers the activation of your full 12-strand DNA matrix which plugs you into your full potential. This is the process.

As we ascend in consciousness toward the love vibration, our ability to manifest with our thought increases. Power of creation peaks when one is living in love; those who are not living in love are less able to manifest precisely what they desire 1) because they simply don't know how and 2) because without this knowledge and the building of their inner love-light they are frankly not very powerful. If we are not motivated by love and creating in love, this power would indeed be dangerous, so this is a useful safeguard. In this way, you might say that such power is kept out of the hands of those who are not ready for it in the same way a sharp knife is kept out of the hands of a 3-year old. It holds amazing slicing power but amazing slicing power in the wrong hands does not a happy ending make. So until we learn to master Love, which starts with removing the genetic contracts and programming that would otherwise misguide our powers, for our own safety and everyone else's, such powers are kept out of reach.

PART II

Activating
Your New Energy Body:
The 12 Sacred Stages

CHAPTER SIX
The Preparation; Stages: 1-4

Stage 1: The New Energy Body Rousing Diet

The reason I address diet as the first stage is because food toxicity is a tangible kind of block. Unlike the emotional and psychological blockages which we will discuss later this one is one you can see, touch and feel.

One of the most important things people need to know about food is that food creates obstruction in the body. Unless it is fresh fruits and vegetables (and their freshly extracted juices) you can be sure it is not energy enhancing, but energy depleting. The role of food is so misunderstood. Everyone thinks food nourishes and gives you energy but it doesn't. The biggest cause of disease is the obstruction food leaves behind as it attempts to pass through the body. The muck it leaves behind in the intestines is absorbed by the tissues and disseminated throughout every cell in the body where it bakes into its new cellular home. This of course, interferes with the critical work the cells need to do and blocks the flow of our inner pathways.

Our physical bodies mirror the flow of the light waves at the root of its structure. Therefore any obstruction in the cell inhibits the electromagnetism in that cell. Eating foods on a regular basis that fill our cells with this obstruction cause a loss of electromagnetism throughout the body at large. Cells lose their electrical force which leads to tissues, organs and ultimately the entire organism losing its electrical force.

We have been so overly-focused on calories, fat grams, carb grams and the like that we have lost sight of what a healthy body is. A healthy body is a body whose cells and pathways are clean and free flowing. When we eat food other than fresh fruits and vegetables (and their freshly extracted juices) our bodies must work very hard to break them down – usually only eliminating part of what we ingest. The rest which we do not eliminate, remains in our body – starting in the intestines where it sits putrefying, creating stagnation in the critical pathway of the intestines. Once this pathway is blocked all others are forced to take on the overflowing traffic of waste until your body is nothing more than a home to a beast of a traffic jam!

You lose sensitivity, you lose power and the stagnation of the congestion goes against everything that life represents – it prevents electromagnetic flow! This, of course, occurs at a different rate with everyone based on their genetic history and the extent of their dietary offenses. But it does happen. The body ultimately will stagnate and create the perfect environment for deterioration and premature death. The waste in the body autointoxicates – meaning the body's poisons kill the body off.

This desensitizing of the body due to improper feeding and elimination makes people unaware of how the body should really feel. A clean-celled body of free flowing inner pathways feels like the light energy wave that it is. The sooner people stop equating food with energy and health the sooner they will understand what creates a perfect human body. The misinformation has been circulating for so long that everyone seems to have taken on their own version of this unenlightened approach to feeding the body. If you still see food as something you should eat three times a day and believe that you need to balance your diet between a certain amount of grain and grams of protein, it is time for a dietary re-education makeover!

The body's fuel is not food stuff or even vitamins and minerals. The body's fuel is electromagnetism. Anything that stands in the way this is detrimental to the body period – this includes vitamin pills, whole grains, animal products, soy products and all the packaged foods that exist. Now, each of these offends the body to a different degree – some less than others. For example raw goat cheese is an animal product, but it is not going to infringe on your electromagnetism as much as a sloppy Joe or deli meats. So, I'm not suggesting that you live on only raw fruits and vegetables. There is room for other foods and it is downright dangerous and, in extreme cases deadly, to stop feeding yourself the poison your body is addicted to all at once. It's a gradual process should you choose to undertake it. The point is just that all the current information that tells the story of non plant food being energizing or healthy in any way is false. Until we accept this we will not get very far in understanding how energy and health <u>are</u> generated.

The important thing for awakening your new energy body is redirecting your intake towards this correct way of nourishing the body and away from the old way. This way, every step you take in this corrected direction will support your electromagnetic truth. With every step toward this new understanding your body will remove more and more of what has been inhibiting it and you will become more and more sensitive to your body as light-energy rather than dense, burdensome matter. It is what comes out of you that makes you healthier, younger looking and more radiantly revivified – not what you put into yourself. The only reason to focus on what you put in is to ensure that you are avoiding the things that would compromise your cellular cleanliness. For example, I love to eat avocados. But I don't' eat them for their vitamins, "healthy fats" or live enzymes. Yes, there are vitamins, amino acids, live enzymes, water and oxygen in avocados. But I don't eat them to get those things. I eat avocados because I like the taste of them and they give me the pleasurable sensation of something creamy and hearty without any drawbacks. You see, because avocados go through the body so quickly and they are a plant food, they leave the body extremely rapidly ensuring that there is no waste (future obstruction) remaining in me after enjoying the pleasure of eating them. You see, I enjoy food. But I know that food is not my sustenance. My physical strength and vitality come from living in a clean-celled body of clear pathways. In this state my body creates everything it needs. Other than fresh air, fresh water and sunlight which I partake of zealously, my clear-flowing, light-energy-waves rich with their Life Force Energy (electromagnetism) ensure my perfect health. When it is time to indulge in food, I am careful not to corrupt that state by eating foods that would detract from my electromagnetic "super-current" (well, most of the time).

I know this sounds radical and maybe even a tad scary. I don't suggest you stop eating today and fast on sunlight and water. That would actually be a really bad idea. What I am saying though is that you can simulate heavier foods and delicious satisfying meals using fresh plant foods that give you all the pleasure without the drawbacks. You can even add some high quality meats or high quality grain products atop this foundation until you feel like taking it to the next level. The only reason it sounds radical is because it is not what is done in our culture. We have been so programmed to believe that food is our sustenance and that we nourish ourselves when we eat hearty portions of hot, dense foods. But remember this always: your real fuel is electrical energy – and you cannot receive the quantities necessary of it if your body is blocked with the obstruction created from unfit foods.

One thing you can do is just cut back on the number of meals you eat. No one into health should be eating three solid meals each day. That's just too much food. You can trade your bagel, eggs or cereal in the morning in for a vegetable juice. That would help tremendously! Also rethink the way you vilify certain foods. Sugar, for example gets a bum rap. Contrary to popular belief, sugar doesn't make you fat – it's the stuff around the sugar – the milk, flour, shortening – that makes you fat. Nobody sits around eating raw sugar cubes! Sugar is mixed into obstructive ingredients and then the sugar gets blamed. This is why foods like sugar free cookies are still so fattening yet eating fresh fruit on an empty stomach in a clean body is not.

While you're at it, don't give the label "organic" more credit than it deserves! That too means nothing. If you think soy or wheat are any better for you if they are "organically grown" you are sorely mistaken. Unfit foods are unfit foods. Here are some other unfit foods to keep away from: yogurt, all pasteurized milk products (which are as life- depleting as beef or pork), anything that is not from a whole food source, sodas, low quality restaurant food, fake cheeses and fake soy replicas of non-vegan foods (that stuff is really scary)! You do not have to eat exclusively organic foods, *but you do need to eat the highest quality food you can find under the circumstances* and avoid all junk and junk disguised as healthy food. Pay attention and look out for purity in anything you are going to ingest. Processed packaged foods will rob you of the experience of your new energy body!

A highly waste-impacted body fogs up the mind, feelings and intuition. The cleaner you can get your cells, the more readily your truths will come through. This is why we start with the body. I want you to be as receptive to all this incredible information as possible. The more of your physical density your can release, the more easily you will be able to intuitively comprehend and grasp the Big Picture of your limitlessness.

A diet rich in Life Force Energy foods with some simple cooked foods in easy-to-digest combinations is the first step to clearing the body enough to prime yourself for this awakening. You don't have to become obsessive about your diet in order to sufficiently cleanse yourself for this awakening. Just try to stick to these four principles:

1: Eat only fresh fruit or fresh fruit or vegetable juice in the a.m. (Fresh carrot juice for example would be perfect.) Avoid fruit and fruit juices if you are in the least bit sensitive to them. If you get bloated after eating fruits, you'll be better off waiting until your body is a little cleaner to enjoy them. Otherwise the fruit is just running into "back-up" in the intestines and further fermenting it causing it to take even longer to digest, making an even more friendly environment for undesirable bacteria and fungus to thrive.

2: Eat flesh with vegetables or starch with vegetables **but do not eat starch and flesh together in the same meal.** Note: the only starches I would recommend are baked root vegetables like starchy squashes and yams or the highest quality sprouted grain or whole grain products. If you eat flesh try to limit your flesh to no more than once a day (preferably at dinner) and stick with low density fleshes like seafood.

3: Avoid overeating on dense foods like starches, nuts, beans; meanwhile EXAGGERATE your portions of very light foods like large all raw vegetable salads and steamed vegetables. (Fruit can be enjoyed for breakfast as long as you are not bloating and as long as you eat them on an empty stomach).

There really is one key concept for dietary success: SIMPLICITY. Most people when they get into raw foods or vegan foods or any other variation on healthier eating, they start looking for recipes and dishes that mimic the stimulation that the heavy foods they were eating before offered them. The goal is to be able to sit down to a simple raw salad with avocado, a couple of baked sweet potatoes or a filet of fresh fish and a head of broccoli and green salad and enjoy that. We must start appreciating simple foods and simple combinations and seeing it not as "diet food" but perfectly normal, every day fare. Anything heavier should be seen as an aberration to this rule – not the other way around. So there you have it. All these theories on diet and all it takes is eating simple, clean, inexpensive, uncomplicated, fresh food. One day, folks will wake up to the enormous inconvenience of "convenience foods" and realize that fresh from the earth food was, is and always will be the most convenient in all ways.

This is not to say that it is wrong or bad to play with more masterful creations in health foods and make gourmet raw dishes, enjoy making new things and such. Many people do this throughout their levels of transition and indeed it becomes very much a hobby for those with a penchant for food prep. All I am saying is that it is unnecessary. For those who are seeking to quickly remove physical waste for a greater plan, who are driven to make more efficient strides with the spiritual part of their lives, over-complicating clean eating can become a distraction. Find a way to create balance in this if utter simplicity is not your thing. Allow what needs to happen for you keeping this knowledge in mind.

An end to mind numbing eating: so many people eat mindlessly because they 1) are not conscious of stored up stale energy and feelings and 2) they don't release these energies to allow the natural flow of fresh, life-generating energy. It always comes down to the free flow of energy -- don't ever forget that!

It is of vital importance to include plenty of grounding foods as part of our daily intake as you proceed with igniting your light body/DNA activation. This doesn't mean you need to consume heavy foods, however including some root veggies like baked sweet potatoes, raw or cooked beets, parsnips or pumpkin/squashes will help keep you grounded as your vibrations increase. It's a good idea to reflect on the vines, roots, systems of connection to earth and each other as you enjoy your plant food. This visual will help ground you. Also, the better you feel in your body the less you will desire escape from earth and the more you will enjoy your physicality as a guidance system and the pleasures of earth.

There is an extensive amount of dietary information on my website as well as of course in my first two books: *The RawFood Detox Diet* and *Raw Food Life Force Energy* (both published by Regan Books/Harper Collins).

Stage 2: Guided Meditation for a Pleasant Awakening

Yogis have taught meditation from time immemorial. To quiet the mind and enter the perfection of inner silence is the gateway to all the answers we seek about our world and our existence. From this place we can become "self realized" as it's often termed. However, we are a culture that spins in the brain at such a rapid rate that it is virtually impossible for modern man to center himself in such a state of peace much less become self realized. This is where guided meditation comes in. It offers a transition from the spinning brain to these ultra-peaceful states. A good guided meditation can help place the reigns of the mind back in the hands of the individual in a gentle, enjoyable way without compromising the ultimate goal of being able to achieve perfect inner peace and higher states of awareness.

When all our energy gets tied up in our heads, we completely lose touch with the resonance of peace. We live in the head going from one out of control trajectory to another and lose touch completely with the heart and our feelings. The male energy of the intellect can spin at incredible speeds and is the force behind our modern routines, drive, ambitions and daily challenges. There is so much we have to do in a day – from organizing our time to managing our careers, in many cases managing other people, parenting children, households and endless other things. All of these tasks take place in the brain – turning folks into mad weavers doing/thinking, doing/thinking, doing/thinking – spinning spinning, spinning! And then we wonder why we have high blood pressure or atrophying skin and cannot be still for a moment without getting fidgety.

We have taken this imbalance to such an extreme that emotional and psychological illnesses stemming from this very madness – things like OCD, Tourette Syndrome, facial paralysis, IBS and myriad symptoms of chronic stress are now commonplace. We have become disordered but we can also become reordered again.

We have also become so dependent on our minds that to "let go and let flow" is a terrifying concept to most.   Many are afraid to leave the slightest thing to natural unfolding and put all their energy into trying to control every area of their life until they completely cut themselves off from their dreams, creativity and anything else that might bring some spontaneous magic into their lives.

I'm not suggesting that you must be ready at this point to completely release your controls and allow life to flow without your "safety mechanisms" (perhaps one fine day you will). However, I do want to emphasize the importance of balancing all this "doing" and "thinking" with equal measures of "being" and "feeling." This can only be done by quieting the "brain chatter" and open to the experience within the body and the pulse of the heart. This is the first step to grounding your being in the body. Being in the body (as well as in the mind) is essential to being able to transmute your material body – carrying it into the higher vibrational states we've been discussing. Getting stuck in the head is oh so common today but it is a trap.

Being and feeling are the ways of the feminine path. This brings life experience into the body where our feelings reside and into the heart where our center can be felt. We would ideally "BE" moment to moment from this place in our hearts. One good exercise is to try to think and lead from your heart center for one day – or even just an hour and observe the immediate difference that living from your heart center instead of your head center makes to your life experience, choices, relationships and energy level.

Utter stillness supports the birth of the New Energy Body whereas a cluttered mind prevents it. When you can stand in the strength of your inner silence whilst all the dramas of life rock and rattle around you, you will have achieved self-mastery. In your silent awareness you will be able to discern what life is really communicating to you through your circumstances and experiences moment-by-moment.

Guided meditation is particularly helpful in this time of head centered living because it goes into the mind to "pick you up" and then takes you somewhere else. By going through the mind it honors where mentally-driven people are. People who start out with strongly imbalanced mental leanings can be equally successful as those who start out in a more grounded heart space if they stick with it. They just need someone to speak their language. In fact, they often become the best students and teachers because they explore the sacred geometries, quantum and cosmic worlds from the analytical side which helps move these teachings from being pigeon-holed as "new age" instead of just being what is.

Personally, the two things that helped me most in terms of activating this new energy in my body were my regular guided meditations with my Almine CDs and the ritual of daily bathing. I am a busy mother with an active business and social life yet this was my quest so I made the time for it. If you really want this you must make the time to do it. If you do it can work anywhere – I'm living proof if I can do it with my schedule in the middle of Manhattan! One thing you might want to keep in mind is that when you eat clean, unadulterated, natural foods and keep your intestines and bowel[7] clear you do not need to spend time in a gym or working out. You can put that hour that you might ordinarily put aside for your exercise routine into this. It will certainly be more pleasant!

When you listen to a meditation from someone who has arrived at self-mastery such as Almine Barton, Amorah Quan Yin, Lee Harris or Story Waters (there are of course others that you may discover on your own), not only do you receive the truth of their words, but their pure love essence which has become so refined and in tuned with the Source's it will awaken your own. You will not just hear words, you will be lifted and tuned into the pure essence that will guide you effortlessly exactly where you want to go (which is to fully develop and live within your own pure love essence and the strength of that stillness).

One of the main reasons people overeat is because they are feeding the body from the intense spinning energy of the brain. Their way of eating is a reflection of their thinking. If they would only take the time to practice some from of mediation before the time of day when they typically binge or enjoy their big meal of the day, they would find themselves eating slowly, and registering when they have had enough. You maybe accustomed to regulating your food intake via intellectual values like calories, grams of fat, protein or food weight. May I suggest rather that as you put the emphasis on creating peace and expanding your vision, you will no longer need to self regulate in this way.

---

[7] The International colon therapy directory is scheduled to be completed and up on my website by August 30, 2007.

Doing a simple meditation before eating helps remove so much of the pressure that causes our weight to balloon. There is a sub-conscious instinct to try to balance out these intensely weighted male-focused energies. But unfortunately many people unwittingly use food to do it. They eat and eat furiously (I call this the "stab and swallow" technique) in an attempt to try to ground themselves back into the body through the feeling of fullness. Of course, trying to ground the body this way is always counter productive and just gets us back into our head – in worse ways because we then start judging ourselves for over eating, for lacking discipline and then dwell on how we are finally going to lose the weight all the while remaining stuck in the vicious cycle.

Bringing conscious awareness into the body, into our cells, our hearts and rooting us in the earth (think of your body as your personal universe's "earth") taps us into the part of ourselves that nurtures, is soft, gentle, feminine and compassionately available to ourselves and others. When we learn how to feel again, safely, we will not need to ignore our deepest needs, numbing them with our addictions or running from them in fear.

Finding the right guided mediation is really important. I would like to recommend the following CDs which are all available via the internet[8]: Almine Barton, Lee Harris, Story Waters and Peggy Phoenix Dubro. These will not only help bring you into an ideal frequency but also help you heal your subconscious and unconscious wounds.

---

[8] Amazon.com, spiritualjourneys.com, emfbalancingtechnique.com

I recommend actually lying down for maximum value in these meditative states. Lying down allows you to go into the deepest states because there is no thought or effort required to hold your body up or discipline yourself in any way. Since your spine is straight when you are laying down you will also ensure that the pranic tube within your spine can pass this new energy through you without obstruction. Expect to feel deeply rested after such a meditative journey!

This approach to meditation fills us up with our "daily bread" of energy-essence. We must do it as regularly as we would take in food. Food is only **minimally** sustaining to our being. Filling up on our inner essence is **maximally** sustaining!

Use the suggested meditations as often as possible, ideally daily. I also encourage you to try a variety of meditation CDs in order to find the ones you best connect with. This stage is fundamental and I encourage you to enjoy this practice as often as possible.

"Matter is like a small ripple on this tremendous ocean of energy, having some relative stability and being manifest...And in fact beyond that ocean may be still a bigger ocean...the ultimate source is immeasurable and cannot be captured within our knowledge." – David Bohm

Stage 3: Awareness of the Ripple Effect

Our body is a living community of cells. Each cell within our body has all the systems and characteristics that we have as a whole: a digestive system, respiratory system, nervous system, lymphatic system, etc. In this way, we can see our cells as a microcosmic reflection of ourselves. We can look at a single cell and better understand ourselves just as we have better understood our world by looking deeply into the subatomic structures of it – the most microcosmic structures hold the imprint of the macrocosm.

What we do to one cell likewise is done to every cell. If we take unnatural food into our body it affects our moods and our work. When we watch and invite violence in our lives it effects our perception, our digestion and our dreams. Like a pebble thrown into a stream has a "ripple effect," we are made of water and we conduct thus through that water; everything that comes into our "sea" throughout the system is affected!

When we think of ourselves as separate from our fellow man, judge harshly or act in hurtful ways, we likewise suffer in our inner life. We develop cancers or fail to achieve things we would like to achieve. Everything we do affects our whole being – the part that we identify with as well as the larger cosmic whole that this process helps us grow to identify more with. When we ingest fresh vegetable juice, reflect on nature, speak from the kindness in our hearts and cherish the divinity in our fellow man our lives likewise reflect that. This is the ripple effect.

In this way you can also see how your body, which is a community of cells, will reflect the state of those cells. If there is harmony in the community there will be harmony in the whole. If there is discontent, there will likewise be disease in the community.

Ever since we have started mapping human DNA we have heard the scientific and medical communities echo that we are at the mercy of our genes (i.e., if we are fat, lazy, prone to certain illnesses, etc. it's because we inherited those illnesses). Wow, what a way to dismiss your personal responsibility, excusing your life away because you claim the heritage of a particularly maleficent gene! You may have been born with certain genetic inclination from the combined chromosomes from your parents, but you can activate and terminate these tendencies as easily as you might select dishes on a take out menu. The ripple effect changes our makeup constantly as we move through different environments, moods, thoughts, jobs and relationships.

Our genetics are determined by more than their physical programming. As our cells renew through the detox process, the genetic codes within our cells will renew, redefining themselves based on what the new cells resonate with – not just with what our cells and genetics were originally programmed to resonate with. We can emphasize different genetic tendencies through adjustments we make to our thoughts, environment and all our choices. The shifting of vibration and focus will shift the tendency and the tendency will shift the outcome. You might say you are managing your own personal genetic engineering project!

This is also why we must move away from perceiving our lives and our dreams in a vacuum. We must take life in its larger context. Seen in its fullness it becomes clear that everything we do affects everything around us – rippling right through. Do you have cancer or are you trying to find a cure for cancer? Well, we must stop trying to fix it in a laboratory – this is the vacuum mindset. The cause of cancer transcends the cancer itself. The cancer imprint took form because the person was exposed to a world where ripples of cancer-creating thoughts, emotions, foods, or other inharmoniously vibrating substances were introduced. Cancer is an imbalance that has its roots in inharmonious living (whether emotional, environmental, dietary, psychological (or all of the above), it is all the same: the cause is a factor of inharmonious vibes pulsating/rippling though the being. The "eagle vision" mindset that sees the ripple effect helps us to see through the illusions of perceiving in a vacuum and therefore offers real solutions for healing.

Take Government for example. If the individuals making the laws and governing the dispensations are not themselves peaceful and harmonious how can the community they govern possibly be expected to be peaceful? If these factions are instead warring, angst ridden, drug-dependent, money grubbing and perceptually compromised, what will such a ripple effect have on the ocean they rule. The ripple effect is a micro/macro cosmic law that operates on all levels and all bodies. This can be used to our great benefit because small drops spread quickly!

Every thought, every bite of food, every interaction we have with one another affects the tendencies of our DNA, our sacred geometric blueprint, our vibes and thus our fate, ergo we ought to pay very close attention to and be much more deliberate with our choices in all these ways.

So you can see that like a rock tossed onto body of water, everything that enters their body ripples through it, affecting every system, organ and ultimately every cell. We are, after all, made mostly of water. But it is also much bigger than that – these ripples move through our larger universal body – our world, solar system and universes!

Stage 4: Aligning with the Breath

The in-breath and the out-breath represent every key part of our world: it is the male/female, the +/-, assimilation/elimination, power/surrender, night/day, contraction/expansion – it is the perfect illustration of what makes life tick, the electromagnetism. The story of the breath connects the highest dimension with the lowest dimensions – from our universe to our cells. It is the pulse of life. To miss aligning yourself properly with the breath is to miss the key conduit of the whole cosmic dance.

The breathing exercise I suggest below will bring immediate peace and energy, reminding us that energy really comes from Life Force Energy/Pure Love Essence, not sugars and proteins. These exercises also massage the internal organs relieving the even the worst stresses.

This is really a revolution in breathing because what I want to suggest to you goes far beyond the concept of inhaling for the sake of taking in oxygen. What we want to do is actually see ourselves in the larger context of the universal body connecting to the Source of all. In this way we see our "signal" coming from a great source of power and then we transmit that power in the exhale throughout our body and into the world. You receive the love energy from the Source and then you transmit it though and beyond yourself flooding your own body with its precious essence and electrifying the space all around you with this vital clear light. I am asking you to breathe the Universe as the Universe breathes you – just as with every breath you can imagine your cells taking in and exhaling the oxygen you send into them as you bring the Life Force Energy into your lungs and skin.

Think about how the ripple effect will carry this into the world at large all because you made the conscious effort to receive and transmit it. What you'll quickly discover is that you go from holding the concept of "receiving/transmitting" into realizing that what it actually means is that you are conducting this energy. You are a conduit through which this energy flows. Along with everything else you do in your life, you can impact the world in such a positive way simply by becoming a conductor of pure Life Force Love Energy!

Breathing exercise for receiving and transmitting universal energy: Close your eyes and bring yourself to a state of inner peace (the best you can muster) to begin. Start to feel the limitlessness around you and imagine that there is a source of power that has created this limitlessness. Find the source. Envision a beam of light moving between that power and you. Watch it grow larger in circumference and more luminous until you feel strongly connected to it. On the inhale say to your self as you deeply draw in a breath, "I am receiving." Feel yourself receiving the voltage of this vitality through the top of your head like it's an antennae and surrender to it so that it can move down through your body through the interior of our spine. On the exhale, say, "I am transmitting." As you do, feel the energy move through you and out of you as though you are generously pouring it out into the world. Imagine the love energy you have contributed to this power as it goes out beyond your personal space and nourishes your surroundings. Open your heart to the love that you can send out. With each breath allow yourself to receive more of this love energy as you inhale and transmit more as you exhale. 21 breaths would be ideal. Eventually, work your way into merging the concepts of receptivity and transmission into the marriage of the two poles of the breath. You can lose yourself in this one thought through each deep inhale and exhale: "I am conducting Love Energy." With practice, this could be your state of being every moment!

When are you going to start breathing properly? When are you going to make time in you life for the one thing you need and cannot support life, much less basic health without?

Focusing on our breath will also help remove the restless brain chatter so that we can enjoy the silence of our essence. When we breathe deeply in a deliberate manor, we make the time to refill with our essence and quite the mind. Quieting the mind is critical, not as an end unto itself, but as a way to stop living in a state of constant distraction and outside stimulation.

After some time of practicing aligning with the cosmic breath, you will graduate to turning life into a walking meditation which means that we remain in touch with our pure essence whether we are driving, shopping for groceries, in business meetings, helping our children with homework and hanging out with our friends. Regardless of what goes on around us, we serve ourselves best by remaining closely aligned with our inner light. You can walk in the inner bliss of stillness moment-to-moment. Simply keep practicing holding the belief that this state of being is entirely possible and you will see it gets easier and easier.

One really important thing to remember with meditation, cleansing diet and breathing exercises is that they are not meant to be an end unto themselves but a way to become more aware and connected. The goal is not to become a great meditator or a great breather or a great eater – the goal is to be in alignment with truth moment to moment. These practices just help us across the great chasm that lies between the old state of being and the new one.

Exercise: Reaching the Aligned State of Being: Allow yourself to take a part of your day to dramatically reduce your pace such that you are functioning at a dramatically slow pace (mentally and physically). You will notice that in this state you do not oppose life in any way but rather you naturally harmonize with life. This requires a deep surrender that you will get better at over time. Start small, by surrendering to just the next few moments or the hour. Higher states require surrender. You can practice by surrendering to a fresh inhale. Allow yourself to surrender to the inflow of breath and watch how much more you are capable of taking in. Power is the opposite pole of surrender which means that they balance and support each other. The more you surrender to your breath, the more powerful you will be. Feel the power that emerges from you as you exhale. It is not in the force of the exhale that you will witness it. That may be subtle. You will witness it in the inner power that will radiate from your core and out through your limbs. Notice how you become sovereign like the SUN, shining forth in all of your glory with no worries or mental chatter as you imagine the world revolving around your perfect, powerful stillness. Here you stand, nourishing all life around you, sustaining your light as a beacon, effortlessly giving life-generating energy, light and warmth to the world around you.

Stay with the concept of surrendering on the inhale and radiating forth (like the sun) on the exhale as you imagine your bright shining energy form rays and dancing light clusters all around you. Move through your day in this light with such attention to each moment that you are able to predict and avoid any oncoming distraction that could potentially veer you off course of this alignment and deplete you of this radiance and focus. Remember, you are the river through which the power of the universe flows. Remain aligned and you will witness your power, energy and essence grow.

CHAPTER SEVEN
The Awakening; Stages 5-8

Stage 5: Embodying your light

The sooner you can start to perceive your world as electromagnetic vibration-currents of energy the sooner you will be seeing things as they are. It's one thing to know that matter is light-energy on an intellectual level but quite another to feel and perceive yourself and the world around you as pulsating waves of light that all blend and move as one giant wave of electromagnetism. For a few of you, yes, this will feel natural but for others it sounds a lot like science fiction! Whatever the case, do your best to work with the image.

As we've discussed extensively, there are worlds up on worlds and expansive as well as contracted perspectives by which we can observe and feel our electromagnetism. For practical purposes let's work within the framework of "world" of our physical body rather than the microcosmic cell, for example or macrocosmic galaxy to the expanded extreme. From the perspective of your body, embodying your light means moving beyond intellectual theory of the concept of your body being electromagnetic light energy waves and actually seeing and feeling your physical unit as a diaphanous wave of light. It is about feeling your body in a new way – as a living flame of electromagnetic energy.

If you have not already created a visual in your mind of yourself as a wave of electromagnetic light, try to do so now. Only when you stop perceiving yourself as some crude material construct and start seeing yourself as pure light can you then embody this great torch that you are and enjoy all that comes with that.

Let's go back for a moment to the Einsteinian model that matter light and energy are one. At the subatomic level, all is oscillating light energy. We are light energy oscillating rapidly with a tremendous amount of life force animation. At its very essence light is FIRE! From the microcosmic perspective, the axis within each atom of each cell is a pole of fire-light; imagine that your spine has a tiny inner-tube running through the length of it. This spinal "core" is the fire-axis which holds your spinal fluid. The essence of this fluid is liquid-light, your inner flame. There is even a name for this "inner tube." It's called your "pranic tube." It is the very electromagnetic core we discussed in chapter three when we explored the primal torus pattern of nature's sacred geometries.

The pranic tube (also known by its Sanskrit term "sushumna") is the location where the Kundalini or Life Force Energy rises up the base of the spine through the various energy centers in the body into the head center. This is your living flame, the coherence of all your life force condensed. Here you can tap into your full aliveness and, it is rumored, overcome aging and even death. We know so little about our bodies really. We have a center for life force! We have a center for everything and all are one in the larger flame of our LIFE LIGHT!

Imagine your body as a living flame whose greatest intensity runs right through the vertical axis of your body. Become aware of the flame's power in the "chakra"[9] centers of your body. Feel the power take hold at the base of your spine in your root, then feel the creative energy alive in the area halfway between the base of your spine (a.k.a. your "root") and your navel; then feel the Life Force Energy awaken in that flame at the spot right behind your navel; next feel your heart center surge with the power of this fire; allow the fire to rise into the throat opening and enlivening that area while you imagine how you can express yourself more authentically in all ways; feel the heat in your forehead as the flame rises inside your brain, between your eyes and then finally allow the flame to surge through the top of your head (your crown), up into the higher realms where it will connect with more spiritual dimensions of your energy field. Notice how your posture naturally lifts, opens and surrenders to the flow of this energy so gracefully as you follow the flame up your spine.

---

[9] Chakras are the seven major vortices on the body's energetic pathways. These vortexes are located in the following places: the base of the spine, three inches below the navel, just behind and slightly above the navel, the heart, the throat, the third eye (area between the eyes, centered on the forehead), and the crown (top of the head). There are many other chakra centers but these are the major ones.

Once you have felt the power of this flame and the route it follows ascending and descending via your spine. Imagine the flame is rising from your base. Rise with it. Notice how it lifts your mid-spine and opens your shoulders like wings; note how your head is drawn back ever so slightly and how you are effortlessly lifted like a swan or a giraffe. Feel your flame rise and emit its powerful energy all around you. Open up to its fullness and embody your power fully. This is our natural alignment. Did you notice that the upward flow of this energy marching up your spine effortlessly and elegantly straightens your posture?

No longer do we need to force our body into a rigid sense of correct posture. That is the way of the old energy body. Instead we gain natural poise by simply allowing the flow of energy to lift us into spinal alignment with the sushumna. Among so many other gifts, embodying your light graces you with perfect posture.

Remember this as often as you can as you walk to work, shop for groceries, type emails. Notice how much clearer and how much more heart-centered your communications and emotions are when you embody your flame.

Fanning your flame

The one thing that best sustains a fire is oxygen. Breathing oxygen-rich fresh air fans our fire-light. As you know, respiration has two parts – the inspiration and the expiration. To inspire is to take in oxygen; to expire is to breathe out carbon dioxide. We take in the life energy and we give away death (expiration) with every breath

Ask yourself this: when you breathe, are you fanning and maintaining a flaming fire or suffocating yourself and your fire with shallow, tiny inspirations. Are you just inhaling minimally? While a balanced inhale and exhale is ideal, did you know that it is most common today to emphasize the exhale -- the expiration? If you are emphasizing the expiration, you must not be surprised if you start to "expire" early. Bring more emphasis to the inhalation and trigger an increase in your pure essence through the fanning of you inner fire and what I like to call the "Life Hormone" (the yet to be medically validated essence that runs through the endocrine system beginning at the pineal gland and running right down to the sex glands) when we are aligned with the Source Light.

What about your diet? Does your approach to food enhance the electromagnetism of your cells and the unobstructed flow of your pathways? Do the foods you eat pour oxygen into your body (all raw fruits and vegetables and their juices are great oxygenators whereas cooked foods and packaged foods are oxygen devoid) or do you put your flame out bite by bite by eating low oxygen foods meal after meal? Taking in oxygen then can be seen as the most primal source inspiration! It's inspiring stuff!

Holding and fully embodying our fire-light is not drudgery like the severity of holding postures and strict organized rules. It is a natural flow that will take you up and out, opening you up and making you feel like a rose blossoming into your fullness!

"Come and listen in to a radio station

Where the mighty host of Heaven sing

Turn your radio on…

If you want to feel those good vibrations

Coming from the joy that his love can bring

Turn your radio on…

Don't ya know that everybody is a radio receiver

All you have to do is listen for the call

Turn your radio on…"

- Turn Your Radio On, Andy Griffith

-

Stage 6: Tuning and Raising your "Light Quotient"

The 3rd dimension is a funny place to be because while there is a lot of knowledge and light to be found here, there is a lot of misunderstanding as well. The light quotient is forever in the balances on earth meaning that by the virtue of free will, we can choose to increase or decrease our personal light quotient.

The process of bringing more light into our bodies naturally transmutes the dark, dense space into light thereby effortlessly changing the dark-density into illuminated vibrant, highly vibrating energy. Every little bit closer to the light you go, the higher your vibrations are raised and the more knowledge you hold in your body.

When we are in our full light we can no longer be directed or controlled by an outside entity "pulling our strings." We become free of the world's dictates and any sense of disempowerment that would otherwise have us marching in step to a drummer other than ourselves. Awakened and aligned we leave the habits directed by fear, commonality and obligation behind. Raising our vibratory rate answers and solves all of these issues for us. The more refined our light, the more empowered we become. Our personal sovereignty and freedom is equal to the light quotient we have aligned with.

When you create an oxygen/Life Force Energy rich environment for your light you will increase it, causing it to grow in power – to glow with more intense frequency. You started building your fire the moment you tapped the big picture in chapter one. Since light is knowledge it will therefore carry more knowledge. Higher dimensions are simply higher states of knowledge/awareness/consciousness. We can all reach these higher states of being by simply raising our vibratory frequency.

Raising your vibrations is a deeply pleasurable sensation and key to awakening your limitlessness. Raising the vibrations of your cells is "ecstasy" – a cellular, emotional and mental ecstasy. This state of being is indescribably pleasing, peaceful and yet thrilling all at once. It warms the heart and eases all earthly distresses from the very first wave of pulsating bliss. Attuning to a higher vibrational energy gives the physical sensation of "quickening" throughout the body but especially in the heart, belly and throat. It fills each cell with a nectar-like essence that feels tingly and blissful. It will feel familiar and thrilling at once.

What I discovered after cleaning my cells of my years of built up toxicity was precisely this. Tapping into the bliss of these intense vibratory pulsations which extended from my cells to the energy field around my body made me see that there was much more power in me than I ever expected to feel in physical form. If nothing else, the hedonist in me wanted to make sure it would continue!

As you may have guessed, eating in such a way that allows for uninterrupted flow of the electro-magnetic current to connect with each cell in exquisite flow, is essential to attuning yourself with life-generating experiences. But there are plenty of non-food ways to immediately raise vibrational frequencies in the body as well – I call this Vibrational Body Tuning (VBT). These include environmental corrections to our living spaces as well as ways to activate the body to produce its own higher vibration energy. These methods are intensely recharging. They will have a distinctly positive influence on everything and everyone around you. The first step in mastering anything is Self mastery which first requires being vigilant enough to sustain your own authentic vibrations without being negatively swayed by other's frequencies. This may seem impossible if you live and work around lots of people but you will see that it is in fact, perfectly achievable.

As you move closer to the light and you experience the energy in your body being raised, you simply begin to transmute suffering into joy. The big picture is indeed that simple. But practically speaking, it takes a very certain course of action to release the darkness and move into the light. Further, knowing what to do is only part of the process. The other part depends on one's readiness to really accept this gracious state of being for oneself. But, for those who are ready and dedicated it can be done and it will be the greatest experience of your life.

Moving into the light is what we all want deep down for we know it takes us closer to home (home, is uniting with the Creator-light from which all things come). But you will experience the familiar tastes of being home with every veil of darkness that you transmute with the light.

Vibrational Body Tuning or "VBT" is a series of methods for raising your life force and feeling that "quickening" in your heart and in cells using your visualization and imagination faculties. Because everyone responds differently to concepts, I've included three different methods below. Find the one(s) that you respond best to and practice them daily. You can do them anywhere and anytime. I find that before rising and upon shutting your eyes at night to be the most effective. A little mid-day or pre-meeting vibration harmonizing is also highly recommended!

1) Close your eyes and imagine the root of your body at the base of your spine. Now run a "grounding cord" from your root deep into the core of the earth reaching down past the crust and magma into the iron-crystal core of the earth. Once you feel the power of the earth energy running up your energetic core, open the gateway to the heavenly energy by way of your "crown" and feel that power flow into your inner core. When the nod to the "Father" and "Mother" are in place, you may go into the sacred space in the heart and simply feel the sensation of pure love energy radiating from the heart center all around you like liquid Light. Stay with this as this may be enough for you at the time. You may also continue with the second way:

2) Go as deeply into this sensation of the heart as you like. You'll find it to be infinite in it's outpouring of your pure essence. There is an unlimited supply of love energy and it is all for you to tap into and enjoy as you desire it. Feel it flow through your inner core into your throat and down your spine, into your organs, into your thoughts and so on until you feel you are fully attuned to this pure love energy. Enjoy the feeling of vastness that will come over you. You will feel like you are HOME. This can be the channel you broadcast and receive the whole day if you choose to. Stay in this frequency and observe how people respond around you. Notice how you start to create a new life scene by scene

3) Imagine your body surrounded by a powerful vortex of energy. Feel the electrical current of that vortex awakening and supercharging the outermost surface of your body. Feel the blissful charge that gives you. Now, add to this a deep sense of peace emanating from the area where your heart is behind your breast bone. Let this feeling penetrate your body extending in all directions from your head to your feet, arms, etc. You should feel warm while stimulated by these blissful waves. Ride this wave of good feeling for as long as you like, being mindful of your breath. **Now focus on these three attitudes and the feelings they evoke: LOVE, PRAISE and GRATITUDE.** Feel the meaning of these words as you mentally repeat them over and over again. These terms are known as the "ascension attitudes" because they literally raise your vibratory rate.

Tip: Don't reject other frequencies that come through as you tune yourself since that will only get you stuck on them and worse, stuck on the frequency of repression and opposition. Allow the pain and it will pass as love takes its rightful place again. Practice. Just practice. It will get easier and easier.

Sound as a Vibration-raising aid

Sound is an extremely useful channel. Since our bodies are made of water, the electricity of our surroundings runs through us so swiftly like an electric current in a pool of water. A few of the right pieces of music can very quickly affect the body with a new current of electromagnetic force. In most cases, inspirational music, classical music and the deep bliss of choir music brings the desired effect. However, there are also times when only hard core rock 'n roll will do. Remember that there will be all different parts of you that will come up and need to express themselves at different times. If frustration, anger, wildness or rebellion are welling up in you, rebel rock might be just the thing to help you "allow" and "accept" those emotions in order for them to be released.

Teenagers are more tuned in than they typically get credit for. They are still clear and honest enough to feel their angst and allow it. So they slam dance, head bang and shake it off by clubbing all night. We should all take a lesson. What do adults do? Repress it, fill themselves with the poison of their angst until it festers into divorce and cancer.   Get your old hard rock music out and let your body and emotions go with those intense rhythms.

Music is a conduit of energy. Sometimes there is a need for drumming/tones other times hard rock is the only thing that will release some deep, repressed memories/energy. Familiar nostalgic songs will bring up emotions that may need to be released. If you feel the need for a certain type of music go with it. Let it in to do its work.

Movement as a Vibration-harmonizing aid

Dancing in all forms is a great way to work though and shake off stale energy so you can resonate with love energy.

Yoga, like dance and other forms of exercise does the job of helping us release stale energies but it also works on the concept of sacred geometry, putting our bodies into positions that enable the re-harmonizing of our cellular and liquid body crystallization.

Attuning with your environment: Nix tv/media/news/stresses to create a cocoon for your awakening. If the energy we bring into our personal life is determined by what we broadcast in that state, the thoughts we have when we are in a state of emoting and reacting to characters' scenarios in a movie, tv show or magazine article effect the same thing. Think about this when you consider what you want to watch and the kind of life you want to tune into.

If you still want to watch violent movies, soap operas and listen to angry lyrics, feel free. It's not wrong to be in a state of low frequency energy. But it should be a choice that you make consciously, knowing what the result of broadcasting such frequencies are.

The aim of this book is not to get you to be "good" it's to get you to be "conscious." Instead of looking at things as "good" or "bad" a more spiritually mature perspective is always to ask yourself where a particular choice falls on the hierarchy of the highest good – your highest good, another's highest good, a society's highest good, etc. This forces you to actually make choices based on what you know about cause/effect continuum as opposed to value judgments that keep us in the "pre-school" of spiritual evolution and absolve us of real responsibility.

All things (all vibrations) are within your sphere of choice. You can explore any part of life and attract all manner of experiences to yourself – pleasurable or hurtful. Just be aware that 1) it is you who chooses and 2) you do the attracting at all times.

A few thoughts to explore:

- Think of your favorite TV show. Feel the scenes in your body. What is the vibration? Is this the vibration you want to feel, send out and attract to your life?

- Take three minutes and only focus on praise, love, gratitude. Feel this in your body. Would you like this to become your natural state of being?

- In the beginning you may have to make a conscious effort but once you start "tuning" into the New Energy Body all the different aspects naturally attune around and within you.

- Attunement to higher states is a one-stop-shop. If you are attuned to higher frequencies of love you will carry these frequencies through every cell of your body affecting every bit of your being and everything around you – improving your relationships, bringing you more insightful thoughts, more inspiring ideas and actually making you smarter because your electromagnetic pulse will be running at full tilt through every cell in your brain!

At first and for as long as it takes for you personally to work through your alchemical process, tuning your body into the desired frequency will be a conscious exercise. But once you become familiar with the sensation of it, you'll be able to attune yourself to very high vibrational states in a blink. Two things happen when you tune in 1) you acknowledge and allow the feelings you hold before attuning and 2) as you allow, you release and tune into with the desired frequency.

If you want a more mundane reason to raise your vibrations consider this: you will be freed of disease and the death vibration. When you hold more light and reach higher vibrational resonances, your energy body no longer supports your defective emotional, physical and personality states. Look at it this way: if your cells are vibrating at 90 MHz it means that cancer cells (which vibrate at 50 MHz and below, coming from states of being created at that vibration)[10] are no longer a part of you.

When you raise your body's vibrational resonance you support life in your body, not death. It really makes you wonder if death is really as inevitable as we think. Predictably, there will always be people who react to the concept of vastly extended life of immortality who are reviled by such a thought, proclaiming, "who in their right mind would want to live forever in this crazy world?" Well,

[10] From research done by Bruce Tanio at Tanio Technologies – the top vibrational research facility in the world.

that's precisely it, when you're vibing high and in states of bliss, life is different – really top notch! In your "right mind" you *would* actually want to live forever. This, by the way, is an excellent litmus test for determining whether or not you are in your "right mind."

In your "right mind" you would be flowing and growing. It's the static life that is so unappealing. Life is not meant to be static. Life is movement. Anything static is contrary to life and does not survive. We have gotten so attached to our patterns that they are stalling us. If we remain stalled we will not survive. As a phase in the larger rapidly, flowing river of life, almost anything is harmless – even becoming temporarily engrossed in materialism is pretty harmless as a brief phase. However, this is not what has occurred. Our societal views, beliefs and ways of living stalled our cultural flow like a steel trap. We can bring the flow back, at least in our own circles simply by recognizing where we have stagnated culturally, thank this period for its opportunities for growth and experience and then move on. This can be done in the midst of playing roles that require us to live and work among materialism, greed and power-hungry societal norms because we are not rejecting others or judging harshly. We are just observing and weighing our observations against what we wish for ourselves and our highest ideals. Instead, we can call out for our next phase and revive the flow of life for all. The alternative is really no longer an option. The old energy way has been in stagnation for so long it hanging on by a thread.

How much do you enjoy your life? You might ask yourself, "What would have change to make me want to live forever?" For me it was the idea of being able to live in absolute freedom from limitations of any kind – to live unrestricted by common physical constraints, with the ability to avoid or transmute pain and suffering if needed. This is, in fact, what we all have the ability to do – become limitless immortals. But the key is that we do not achieve this state through death as our modern religions suggest, but through life! We are fully capable of being in this transmuted form now – we simply need to tune into the frequency, raising every cell of our physical body into the highest vibrations of love energy – as the song says, "Turn your radio on!"

Stage 7: Releasing Emotional Pain for Reconnection

Now that we have come so far, releasing pains that we have been holding involving experiences, other people and even resentments toward ourselves can now be addressed. The source of most emotional pain (such as depression, anxiety and repressed anger) is _JUDGEMENT_. Other than misguided diet, our self-judgment (as well as our judgment of others) is at the core of almost all of our emotional pain. In a few simple steps we can learn to escape excessive judgment and release our most deep-seated anger and hurts, thereby opening ourselves to healthier, happier relationships and self-acceptance.

Did you know that judgments directly affect your breathing pattern? Newborns breathe full breaths of ideal cadence. I suspect judgment (the sense that we are being judged and the nerve-wreaking aspect of that judgment) to be a the core of our inability to breath freely and fully as adults. You see, when we feel the burden of expectations placed upon us coupled with the concern that comes with the abandonment that ensues when we fall short of those expectations, it's no wonder we stop being free to breathe naturally and fully. If you child or a child that you care for is asthmatic or nervous natured, in addition to considering the mucosal component of their diet, please consider their fears of abandonment due to falling short of expectations or dis-inclusion by the "tribe." Embrace their natural essence and encourage their authenticity and watch all such symptoms disappear as you do. Stop "buying into" the common judgments and you will stop being judged as well. This is the meaning behind Jesus' quote, "Judge not lest ye be judged." It's awfully liberating to all involved.

Imagine the human race is a giant body and this giant body made up of all these people is you (because everything is you). Think of all the people you know as living in the form of limbs and organs within that body. Imagine that one of them has hurt you (abused you in some way, stole something of value, embarrassed you, etc.) Now, you have been walking around with this anger. But this anger is directed at some part of your body. Say your anger is directed at your father; your father is your "leg." Are you going to be any better off by slugging yourself in the leg or stabbing your leg? When we want to hurt those that have hurt us, despite our seemingly obvious rational, it only makes the wound worse.

I personally think the easiest way to forgive others is to remember that what offends you about them it is not actually the essence of the person. You are not really reacting to them (their true nature) at all. What you are responding to are their programs, their history, the way their being has been shaped (or rather dystrophied) by the social, emotional and physical environment that they have been exposed to.

You are seeing what they have taken on from the world, not what they really are. Always try to keep in mind that what you know to be "them" is not actually their authentic self, but a manipulated being taken far, far out of its essence and this will enable you to forgive instantly. Take any human being on the planet that you have a problem with and notice that the things you dislike about them or hold them accountable for in your life are not their true essence at all.

What we rage against in others (until we understand the use of what they teach us by offending us) is what they have been exposed to and therefore represent. Hating others' behaviors is as ludicrous as shouting at a mirror for reflecting. If we are reviled by what we see reflected by our societal norms it is our cue to change it. To perpetuate the same effects and yet curse the result is madness. Everyone around us holds up a mirror of what we are, what we've created or what we support in some form.

This makes it so much easier to love everyone, doesn't it? Those who enter back into their pure essence (as you are doing) go through a process of seeing all the ways in which they were acting out such programs too and recognizing how much of what they were reflecting was not them but their conditioning. How can you hate someone who just didn't know any better? It's as ludicrous as a 12th grader condemning a kindergartener for not being able to read.

Once you see this clearly you can easily send love from your essence to theirs and the disempowering cords can be dissolved. A wave of peace follows and you will be amazed as the relationships in your life and old wounds miraculously heal.

Use this approach for yourselves too when you are the one you need to forgive. So you did some unenlightened things in the past? You were simply acting out your programming. Now you see that programming for what it is and you ditch it, tear it to shreds and walk in your essence more and more every day. This is the real meaning of repentance. This is the only way to let go of the past and be renewed. It's a wonderful and liberating thing to finally see where all our misguided behaviors and attitudes come from.

One important point to remember is that you must be our careful to discern between detox emotions and current pain. Just like when you cleanse the body and detox through your skin in the form of a rash or pimples, these detox responses are not due to new poison you put into your body. They are just the route of departure for the old poisons. Likewise, the depression, moodiness, anger, etc that you may feel as you clear your body of food and emotional waste matter, are usually the old emotions moving out of the body. See it as that, allow it to flow and watch it leave you. Then fill that space you have made by clearing out the old energies with love, praise and gratitude.

If you can't get past yesterday, how are you ever going to be here to get your presents today? What future can you possibly have? Think about it. What are your top 20 judgments? Here are some common ones that might help jog your mind:

- Physical appearances: do you mentally review and criticize or praise other's appearance or clothing?

- Social/economic status: do you mentally categorize people by their social and economic status?

- Education: are you an education snob? Do you think someone is less worthy if they have not received a university degree or greater? Do you revere those who have achieved a certain academic level for that reason alone?

- Age/experience: do you assume things about individuals based on what you know about their age and experiences?

Do these judgments serve your growth? Do they serve the growth of your fellow man? Will they seem as antiquated as Apartheid or segregation in 50 years? Would you be proud of them if they were pointed out publicly?

Your emotional guidance system

Just like illness in the body, emotional imbalances tell us that we are out of balance in our "emotional body." We must consider the ways that our living, thinking, relating and feeling (or suppression of feeling) fail to serve our highest good. Of course, emotional imbalances can also be caused from unfit foods. Usually there is much to harmonize in all these areas but once addressed, just like physical imbalances, a beautifully emotionally balanced person emerges leaving no further need for the pain alarm.

"To JS/07/M/378) **This Marble Monument Is Erected by the State**
He was found by the Bureau of Statistics to be
One against whom there was no official complaint,
And all the reports on his conduct agree
That, in the modern sense of an old-fashioned word, he was a saint
For in everything he did he served the Greater Community.
Except for the War till the day he retired
He worked in a factory and never got fired,
But satisfied his employers, Fudge Motors Inc.
Yet he wasn't a scab or odd in his views,
For his Union reports that he paid his dues,
(Our report on his Union shows it was sound)
And our Social Psychology workers found
That he was Popular with his mates and liked to drink.
The Press are convinced that he bought a Paper every day
And that his reactions to advertisements were normal in every way.
Policies taken out in his name prove that he was fully insured
And his Health-card shows he was once in a hospital but left it cured,
Both Producers Research and High-Grade Living declare
He was fully sensible to the advantages of the Installment Plan
And had everything necessary to the Modern Man,
A phonograph, a radio, a car and a Frigidaire.

Our researchers into Public Opinion are content

That he held the proper opinions for the time of year;

When there was peace he was for peace when there was war he went.

He was married and added five children to the population,

Which our Eugenist says was the right number for a parent of his generation,

And our teachers report that he never interfered with their education.

Was he free? Was he Happy? The question is absurd:

Had anything been wrong, we should certainly have heard."

- W. H. Auden "The Unknown Citizen"

Stage 8: Detoxing Your Detrimental Programming

Awakening your New Energy Body is dependent on how effective you can be at finding and eradicating the programming you have been encoded with. This is where we finally get to address and release the old social programming that has been directing our lives. Once we learn to identify these programs and patterns we can start to override them and direct our choices from our truth rather than from imposed old ways of thinking that no longer serve us. This is the ultimate liberation because it frees us to be authentically ourselves rather than being robots merely carrying out functions that we are programmed to carry out. The detrimental patterns are the ones that recall our robot-self instead of our authentic self.

Think of this as a treasure hunt: every programming you find that no longer serves you is a treasure. So let's go a-program-hunting! Let's start with the most commonly held programs that you may have genetically or socially inherited.

Here are some common ones you can start by slaying:

- You have to work hard to make money
- No pain no gain
- You have to diet and labor in the gym to be slim
- You look older as you get older
- People who are rude to you deserve your vengeance
- You have to be a college graduate to deserve respect
- Sex is dirty

What is proper? What is not proper? We have so many opinions about this but do we really believe them when we hold them up to the light of truth?

How do these programs resonate for you now? Do they "ring true" or are they like a heavy uncomfortable weight that can now be discarded? How would it feel to rip these contracts in your genes up and burn them, clearing your body, you emotions and your mental slate of them completely!

Here's a great method for uncovering and releasing old programming

Amorah Quan Yin gives us excellent direction in her book, *The Pleiadian Workbook* (Bear & company, Rochester, VT; 1996), for canceling old contracts that are inhibiting our authenticity and holding our essence hostage.

The main things required in order to clear a belief are:

1. *Awareness of the belief*

2. *Willingness to acknowledge your belief as a belief and not the truth*

3. *Willingness to let go of the belief*

4. *Willingness to feel and release associated emotions*

5. *Acceptance of the responsibility for creating your own reality and not being a victim*

6. *The ability to imagine an unlimited healthy alternative to the belief*

7. *A method for releasing the old belief"*

Amorah suggests several approaches for canceling these contracts and programs we have accepted. The one that I like the best goes like this:

1. *Get into a place of peace where you feel grounded*

2. *Close your eyes and envisioning the belief (and all the beliefs that go with it) as a pile of contracts, place that pile of contracts that look like stakes of official manila files onto the palm of your hand. Look at the stack and note it's size.*

3. *Take a huge, inter-dimensional stamp in your other hand that reads "CANCELED" and stamp the top of the stack. Imagine the "canceled" stamp burning through all the files.*

4. *Tear the papers up and throw them in a huge bonfire to your right.*

5. *Know it is done. Feel yourself freed of those false beliefs. This may seem imaginary to you if you are not used to trusting this kind of work. But if*

your heart is in it you will be amazed how over time you see these old
beliefs have no further sway over you!

You could do this every time you begin your meditations and in a week burn through a lot of old contracts.

Note: I would like to credit Almine Barton for her in depth teachings on the following information on the "sub-personalities. It was her work that educated me about these "sub-personalities" and how to bring them into harmony for full self-sovereignty. You can learn more about this subject by reading her books and listening to her lectures, all of which are available on her website:
spiritualjourneys.com.

CHAPTER EIGHT
The Fulfillment Stages 9-12

Stage 9: Strengthening the "sub-personalities" to develop emotional sovereignty, inner balance and true Self-reliance

There are four key sub-personalities of our "inner world" that need to be brought into balance before we can expect our "outer world" to reflect balance:

1. The Inner Child

2. The Inner Nurturer

3. The Inner Sage

4. The Inner Warrior

When any one of these is out of balance everything in life falls out of balance. Bringing these four facets into balance is like having all four wheels of your car turning.

Think of these four aspects of yourself as your "inner family." Our inner family is our first level of support and when it is in balance we are completely self reliant – we can say and mean that most powerful statement: "My being is my sustenance."

When we can honestly say and mean this we will have accessed the ultimate joy and peace because we have all the tools to remain fully nurtured, in bliss – fully aware and alive. True joy comes from being in a fulfilling relationship with our self and **our inner family**. Any relationship with another when we are in this space is a preference/enhancement rather than a need/substitute for what we are missing and what needs we would like another to fulfill for us.

When our first relationship is a self-reliant one with our inner family we can finally trust that we will no longer be attracted to dysfunctional people and situations. If we are whole we will attract that which is whole. On the other hand, when we are needy –we will attract those who wish to control because they are also needy.

OUR INNER FAMILY = OUR INNER WORLD

Our relationships with others (our outer family/world) are the mirrors of what we are (our inner family/world).

Let's take a look at the characteristics of our Inner Family's traits when they are in balance:

The Inner Nurturer

Imagine the inner nurturer as the inner mother. When in balance she loves and gives. The nurturer supports growth. She shows a road to growth that does not need to include anything hurtful in order for the growth to blossom.

The Inner Child

The inner child is about five years old. When in balance, this child in you is full of spontaneity and pure innocence. The balanced inner child lives deeply immersed in the moment – seeing through the eyes of the moment – observing every detail and sensation. When the inner child feels safe, loved and free to express it is full of wonders, hearing songs and envisioning magic. Without a happy, expressive inner child, our lives become barren. We lose the ability to have fun. When a balanced inner child expresses sadness it indicates to us that something is not right.

The Inner Elder

(aka the "sage" and the "grandfather") sees behind appearances, listens to input, is wise and interprets the feelings of nurturer and child in order to bring forth it's conclusions which guide the inner family. It gives guidance to the child and nurturer. It governs the nurturer ensuring the nurturer stays in balance. The Inner Elder sees symbolically, meaning that if something happens in our lives it will tell us why that happened and point out what in our lives is out of balance that required this thing to happen so that we could reflect on what needed to be changed or dealt with. Opposition becomes an ally in this way. Things that go wrong in our lives become like a beacon for what needs to be adjusted.

The Inner Warrior

The Inner Warrior defends the "inner family's" boundaries by eliminating or slaying anything that is not supportive of self empowerment. He roots out anything that denies us our truth or threatens our energy-essence supply (such as distractions from keeping focused on maintaining a strong inner flame at all times.) He guards and protects our boundaries, particularly the thoughts that we think which are so critical to the experiences we create. He has "eagle vision" and in this way sees beyond other birds, rises above the occasion creating objective larger vision/perspective.

Now let's look at what happens when the Inner Family falls out of balance:

<u>The Imbalanced, Dysfunctional Inner Nurturer</u> is strict and judgmental which stifles the growth and confidence of the Inner child.

<u>The Imbalanced, Ill-nurtured, Inner Child</u> reacts from its neediness – it looks outside of itself for love, thus clinging to anything that looks to offer some kind of the support and love it has been denied. It also becomes controlling which can be expressed in tirades and tantrums all due to its underlying need to find a

parent where there is none. Your child cannot be parented by anyone other than its own family.

While you may not have had a well-looked-after inner child or free-spirited love-filled childhood, you can give your "inner five-year-old" a good childhood NOW. When the child is parented by his "inner family" it can finally be rocked, comforted, heard and played with and gain all that goes with having had that experience – even if it comes 30 years after childhood!

Those who have not yet had children would be well advised to ensure their inner child is fully functional and joyful before they go on to have their own children. All will benefit greatly!

The Imbalanced, Dysfunctional Elder can be easily spotted because he judges harshly rather than discerns. The role of the inner elder is to discern what is life enhancing and what is not. If he starts judging instead, the family will lose their way. For example, if the inner elder criticizes the inner family for ills that have befallen them such as being evicted from their apartment or having a bad romantic relationship instead of helping the inner family to see the deeper meaning behind why these things may have occurred based on what their thoughts or ways of living and thinking may be attracting, the inner elder will only contribute to further failings for the family in the future. If there is no one to see the deeper vision through discernment, then there is no effective leader and things are doomed to deteriorate further from here.

An Imbalanced Inner Warrior is a threat to the well being of the inner family as well as the community. He gets aggressive and misplaces his anger. Road rage is a great example of an imbalanced inner warrior. He's pent up from having had ineffective boarders so his rage over all that has crossed those boarders sits on the surface of his emotional body ready to rage out on someone or something completely unrelated to the true origins of his anger. An imbalanced inner warrior concedes to programmings of fear, illness, rapid aging, vengeance, jealousy and all other painful emotions because it fails to guard the mind against these and, in its immaturity, winds up fanning them with his red hot rage. In the case of a personal who has been programmed to suppress such emotions there is the risk of blowing out the system internally. The liver is the seat of anger so this organ usually suffers first. In addition to his organ holding the vibration of this person's anger, I suspect this is also behind the imbalanced inner-warrior's sub-conscious self-sabotage of the liver through drinking, drugs or very high fat, toxic foods. When the inner warrior loses focus the protector of the inner family is lost and left in a most undesirable, vulnerable position.

The sub-personalities are not only found in an individual body system. They are found in groups too. You could, for example observe a country's sub-personalities. Unfortunately, with so much wisdom (elder) lost and the nurturing element absent, what we typically see nowadays is a country suffering from a dysfunctional warrior. The "gang" mentality is a great example of a dysfunctional warrior within a group consciousness's inner family. Groups, be they young people entering into street gangs, the Nazis and even society gangs (people of influence who are always trying to stake their various claims) to those who go unguided by their inner elder and uncared for by their inner nurturer wind up fighting outside of circumstances. They bully and fight to own boundaries out of fear for their protection rather than protect their inner boundaries with the eagle vision the elder would have taught them would the elder were balanced. In the case of the latter, there would be very little occasion for asserting their strength or wielding their arms. Groups who are sovereign are naturally peaceful.

Aggression comes from a combination of lack of leadership from the male pole and lack of affection from the female pole. Children raised without these all-essential foundations grow into dysfunctional warriors and tend towards a gang mentality.

Autoimmune diseases are the result of a inner family of dysfunctional sub-personalities on a microcosmic, cellular level. If the governing body is not discerning between what is life-generating and what is life-depleting and the inner nurturer does not care for the cleanliness and nourishment of her family's cells then the cells are going to grow from under-nourished, under-guided cells into fully developed warrior cells fighting each other out of context, angrily pitting cell against cell in a cannibalistic fashion.

Questions such as: What should I eat? How should I care for myself? How should I express myself? Should I be spending my time on this or that? What should I do about this abusive relationship, this career, etc., all seem ridiculous from this perspective. If you are in balance and listening to your inner family the answers are obvious. The balancing of the inner family enables us to trust ourselves and our inner knowing. What this tells us is that we _can_ actually fully trust ourselves – but only if and when we have balanced of our inner family.

Instead of being dysfunctional we can enjoy the highly sought after experience of self sovereignty. Self sovereignty in relationships sets the stage for _interdependence_ – the ideal adult relationship.

While Independence is usually heralded as the ultimate goal, the trouble with independence is that it removes opportunities for personal and communal growth. We do not grow when we simply come to depend on ourselves. While independence is sometimes a critical juncture on the road to interdependence, we must move beyond the stagnation of independence if we are to live in a life-generating way and dance the dance of self-sovereignty in the active world – interacting closely with others in all types of relationships.

Practice honoring your sub-personalities each time you have a difficult issue or emotion you're not sure what to do with. Take the issue first to the warrior and see where he may be allowing negative thoughts into his domain unprotected or fighting out of context. Then take it to the inner sage and see how he would discern the situation and the surrounding feelings or events. Third, take it to the inner nurturer and see what she would suggest to help support a positive outcome and finally see how the inner child is reacting – in a whining tantrum or with innocence and observance out of creativity.

Stage 10: Take up Your Wand!

At this stage we take the understandings about the universal laws of creation from the classroom of Part One into the world and practice what we now know. Recall the two key laws of creation: the first being that (based on the universal law of affinity as explained on page 52) thought and feeling combine to form our worlds, attracting what we send out in the form of our thoughts and feelings which together take on a vibratory note that calls out for the specific thing or experience we request.

Recall that at the end of chapter four, it was suggested that you clear out the muck of your inner programming before you undertaking conscious creation to ensure that your new creations were coming from a pure place of highest good. Recall the reasons that purity is important: 1) creation is more effective and efficient where there is pure intent and 2) you would be more likely to create things of benefit to the whole rather than in a vacuum ignoring the ripples of the micro/macrocosmic effect.

Now, here at stage 10, you are well on your way to clearing your most offensive programming and ready to take up your wand and enjoy the honor of consciously co-creating with the Universe. Consider yourself initiated. You may now pass "Go." Just review the Universal laws governing creation:

Co-creation tips to review:

1) While the power of thought is very strong, the power of emotion is even stronger because it creates the feeling which creates the thought (in

other words, emotion is the driving force behind feeling and thought). But remember: one thing is even stronger than emotion – that is **belief**. Our beliefs precede even our emotions. For example, if we believe it is sorrowful to lack a car, a house and a regular income, we will tell ourselves to feel sorrow if we do not have these things. That sense of lack will create more lack because that is the frequency we are broadcasting. So if we want to change our circumstances, we actually have to change our beliefs.

2)   A couple of prayers spoken or affirmations in the day among the sea of your emotions that you broadcast constantly are not going to make a dent in terms of changing your reality. Be in a walking state of belief in this thing you are creating so that you are broadcasting the signal for it as strongly as possible. This is the difference. Then and only then can things start to change. "Would it be the thoughts of the day or the hastily murmured words at night...whatever our most prevalent thoughts are, they are our most sincere prayers. Prayer is the heart's most sincere desire."[11]

3)   Remember you choose everything. Our life before conscious creation is like a cage. Once we learn that we have the key to our own cage, we can let ourselves out. The key is our beliefs. A new belief can become a new cage or it can become complete freedom from all cages. Therefore think carefully upon what you truly believe and be very wary of anything that does not bespeak of your limitless nature! It is so common for

[11] Almine Barton, from: *The Mystical Keys of Manifestation.* An audio production available through spiritualjourneys.com

people to wish to change their circumstances -- they resent their loneliness, their job, their living space, etc. -- meanwhile if their beliefs, thoughts and emotions were not constantly supporting those things the circumstances would change to reflect whatever those thoughts and beliefs were supporting. It's like saying that we don't want the dinner we made for ourselves or despising the lipstick that we ourselves put on our lips.

4) Manifestation is actually the experience of energetic levels that reside in higher octaves around us taking form by "stepping down" dimensionally into matter and experience.

5) Beliefs create emotions that create thoughts which create feelings which carry a vibration. Once the vibratory note is sounded, atoms are attracted to and take the shape of the geometric blueprint held by the light pattern within the vibration broadcasted from the thought/feeling of its origin. The blueprint of that feeling (held together by its specific geometric structure) is then attracted to atoms which when bonded together in this cosmic magnetism take the form held by the vibration and gives BIRTH to a 3-D structure or experience. This is the cycle.

6) Add the emotional frequency of **Love, Praise and Gratitude** to everything you call out for. This is as essential as the belief that shapes your thoughts because, when you embody (and thus broadcast) the incredibly powerful energy of these three concepts you are acknowledging the core belief that sustains your ability to create in the first place which is that you are the <u>love</u> that can create thanks to the universal laws of the universe which we must <u>praise</u> and be wholly

<u>grateful</u> to for the situation we are in as beings who can do this. This is the belief that feeds every thought that enables your conscious creative ability. We must sustain this belief and broadcast the vibration of it constantly. It is the same vibration as our inner-essence (our flame, our essential being-ness). There is also another reason to focus on these three concepts when we consciously create: the more love-energy we embody, the more power that will be behind our creativity. Hold the love, praise and gratitude trinity of energy in yourself and watch that as it grows so too will your ability to manifest all that you desire.

7)   **Be specific when you create.** Since you will manifest a vibration that holds a specific blueprint for that thing you want, you must be as specific in the visions you hold as possible. For example, if you desire a mate, a man for example, many men may come into your life. But if you are not specific about the type of man you want, you will not see any of these men as the mate you called out for because they are simply not mate material for you from what the cosmos is picking up from your beliefs.

Be precise or your life will reflect the vagueness of your thoughts. If you dream of your future home, for example, send out clear pictures and vibe with the energy you want that home to embody energetically as well as physically or you may get a home but not the home your really want. Don't just focus on having a home but fill it with the vibe that you want to feel in the home, the people you want to come through your home, the kinds of experiences you wish to enjoy. The blueprint makes it possible to include material and non material details because both are essential to designing the experience we seek. The magic is that you can have as much specificity put into your manifestations as your imagination can come up with. Now, do you see why vaguely calling out for a better life, a better mate or better experiences don't result in manifestations that thrill you? Now it may seem like a lot of work to manifest your life but really its as easy as holding the ascension attitudes of love, praise and gratitude because if you are in a state of harmonious vibrations everything you attract will be beautiful and for your highest experience. Like anything new, there's a learning curve. Once you get the "theory" down on your human instrument you'll be able to play "by ear."

8) To change is to thrive; to stagnate is to become obsolete. We cannot expect to change our circumstances unless we are willing to change ourselves. If we want good things to flow like a great job, a great relationship, etc. we need to change our beliefs and our visions. For example, we cannot expect to receive prosperity in our work life if we're still grumbling over our boss and our paycheck. This does not bring for the things resonating with the vibration of joy , pleasure and abundance. In this way we have to manifest from joy, gratitude and love. **Many want things in their lives to change but they are afraid to change themselves.**

"Life is a mirror and that which is within will most certainly manifest without...Thus the warrior changes his world by changing himself."
- Almine Barton[12]

9) You strengthen what which you give your attention to which reminds us that we must take responsibility for manifesting things we don't like that appear in our lives. Somewhere there is something that still needs working on and refinement by our ego so we have called it to us. This point also nullifies victimhood. No one is a victim of anyone but themselves since it is the beliefs of the individual or the group to attract the experience. In this way, we take up our wand when we accept our responsibility to self-govern and the importance of being good stewards of ourselves. When we govern ourselves approach life actively instead of passively, we give up the compulsion to lay blame under any circumstances. This is what separates the wheat from the chaff...most people do not want to accept responsibility even if it means that by doing so they can create a much more exciting, beautiful and fulfilling life for themselves.

I recommend asking yourself at this point the following:

- Am I willing to stop blaming so I can accept the great honor of taking up my wand?

---

[12] Almine Barton, from: *Emotion* (an audio production available through spiritualjourneys.com).

- Can I trust myself?
- If not, what stands in my way?

If something comes up, go out and deal with that thing and then, come back and accept your destiny. Don't worry about being perfect initially. At some point you have to jump in and swim. All you can do is be as vigilant as possible – a good shepherd of your thoughts and subsequent actions.

Stage 11: Sex Re-education

All the things that are out of balance in our lives are carried into our sexuality. We bring the excessive mental focus, our judgments, our fears, our pain, anger, perspectives and subconscious projections into our sex life. If you don't think of yourself as having a sex life (and you are an adult), remember that you cannot separate your sexuality from your larger life experience. Your sexuality is a part of you whether you are engaging with another person or not. Everything you do is a reflection of your sexuality because life is the great dance of the male and female charges interacting inside of us and outside of us every moment.

In the same way that our mental (male) energies have been overworked, imbalancing our feeling (female energies), there has been a brutal split between the physical expression of the male and female union both in and out of the "bedroom."

But let's start "in the bedroom." Meta-physicist Leonard Orr describes sexuality as, making love with the intent of sharing love and human warmth: "sex is spiritual purification; the goal of sex is not reproduction, but human warmth, affection and love."[13] Balance of sexuality attracts its balanced partner and it is here that the most powerful expression of sexuality and the most ecstatic union will be found. Both will become better lovers as a result of awakening their inner essence. Look out for The New Energy Body match-making service coming soon (just kidding!).

If you want the tone of love and connection in sex, you must first embody that yourself. Attune your surroundings and inner experience. Carry this attunement through your voice and your touch, your thoughts and the openness of your heart. Eventually, though it may take time, your partner will likely tune in. The power of this attunement is enormous. Do not underestimate it. Our sexuality and sexual experiences are as much in our ability to mold as anything else.

Our sexuality is a big part of us. It is the part that connects us to our creativity, our passion, our fertility. It is the physical and energetic part of us that ignites our Life Force Energy. When we are out of balance in this area, it affects every other area.

Our sexuality becomes a mirror of our healing. Since it synthesizes all that we believe, feel and represent, when we quiet the spinning mind and experience and acknowledge our love essence, the way we express ourselves sexually is bound to be more natural, loving, nurturing and a more mutually-energizing experience.

---

[13] Leonard Orr, *Physical Immortality*, pg. 55

Media, "Mojo" and Fertility

When two people come together physically, emotionally or socially in the madness of their spinning minds instead of from a state of inner balance and peace, the interaction will only reflect this cacophony. We cannot open to each other like lotus flowers and surrender to overwhelming surges of bliss if we are physically tense and carrying the madness of the day. Yes, some release and pleasure may be better than none at all. And, who, you might ask is going to take the time to ground themselves, release their anxiety and ensure they are coming into the union without any judgments directed inwardly or outwardly? Well, not many. But you, at this next-to-final stage, having learned to attune yourself and master that state throughout your day by regular practice of the other sacred stages will naturally be able to access this state at will. As each of you brings this into your unique relationships, the energy will be heightened and ripple through the consciousness of the masses. Besides, even though it may not be something that everyone decides to do, if you have a strong desire to experience enlightened sexuality, you should go for it! Finally, in short, the pleasure, connection and experience will prove well worth the exercises that precede it.

The irony is that sex is everywhere (I'd love to know what Samuel Taylor Coleridge would have to say about that) and used to sell everything but when it comes down to it, despite what we think, our generation is not sexually liberated. If it were truly sexually liberated we would not be dealing with an issue that has its roots in sexual repression and confusion. What we have is an in-your-face parade of body parts and intercourse which we are told to think of as sexy. The same products that are being sold by way of sexual innuendo are the very products that deplete our mojo – I'm sure you see the irony in this. I cannot tell you how sexually revived couples and individuals become who clear their inner pathways and outer lives of the rubbish that's been holding them down! The old energy way is downright unsexy when held up in comparison to the new energy way.

The growing trend of low natural sex drive tells us a lot about the state of Life Force Energy in the Western world. A low sperm count equates to low Life Force Energy, What all sufferers from "slow swimmers," low sperm count and erectile dysfunction need to know is that their issues are directly related to the extent of obstruction of Life Force Energy in the body. What's creating this obstruction of Life Force Energy? All the things we have discussed so far that must be changed: difficult to digest foods, emotional and mental stressors, inharmonious vibrations in your sphere and poor, shallow breathing. A man's natural sexuality is an excellent mirror of his cellular and intestinal cleanliness.

If it is, shall we say, "falling flat," this clearly indicates that the man's life force is down, way down. What are we planning on generating life with if not life – yet our bodies are riddled with death, disease, sluggishness, fatigue, stress. Do you seriously think these things are going to create a human being – do you seriously believe your chances are any greater if they are swirled around in a Petri dish in the life-force-energy-devoid environment of a hospital or laboratory?

Since our sexuality and Life Force Energy are so interrelated, it makes sense that with the disintegration of sexual health and sexual expression in our culture (due to all these imbalances and misguided messages in the media regarding sex), both fertility and virility are significantly on the wane!

There is an obvious and critical connection between the global infertility crisis and decline in Life Force Energy in modern man. A female who doesn't have adequate Life Force Energy in her body, flowing through her womb will not be able to conceive. Life begets life. Lifelessness does not produce life (no matter how it is manipulated). Think about it. A man or woman living on minimal amounts of Life Force Energy is not going to have life force infused seeds or eggs to fertilize or be fertilized. This applies to his procreation as well as natural sex drive. The state of our cultural "mojo" and the infertility crisis are directly linked. In this way, developing The New Energy Body can be seen as an excellent an alternative for would-be-parents who would like options to fertility drugs and medical intervention.

For life to come forth we need a seed full of the masculine Life Force Energy. We also need a void from it to "spring" from – healthy, life generating female "soil." If either of these things does not exist or is low on life force or fecundity, nothing will spring forth. You wouldn't sew seeds on a rock or expect a harvest to manifest without planting. Without life force within us we will undoubtedly grow more infertile every year, as individuals and globally.

Fertility issues affect at least one in six couples in the United States. This statistic means that every month more than 7 million U.S. couples experience the pain and disappointment of failing to conceive. (The American Fertility Society states that a couple is considered infertile when pregnancy has not occurred after one year of coitus without contraception). [14]

Fertility is ripe, juicy and vivacious -- not exhausted, stressed, over-worked, angry and resentful. Are you fertile, all things considered?

Stage 12: Seeing with Eagle Vision

This final stage finds us at the peak of the pyramid with a solid foundation for expanded perception. From here we can be the conscious designers of our lives that we were designed to be.

Stage 12 is the stage of EAGLE VISION. From the eagle's perspective you lift yourself up and out of the limited view from the ground and you can see the whole of the landscape below. When you see with the eyes of the eagle you can determine what is actually occurring without anything obstructing your sight. You can see the tapestry unfold below in the 3rd dimension in a way you could never see it from your restricted point of view in the herd. When you're in the herd, it's just not possible to see everything as it is from way up above where the picture tells a very different and much clearer story.

So whether it is your diet, career decisions, relationship issues or any other choice you are navigating, pull yourself up and out and see with eagle vision what is going on below.

---

[14] The American Fertility Society

If you are tempted to eat a cheeseburger and fries, pull out and up and look at your body with eagle vision and see what the ripples of such a choice will manifest through your body and state of mind. When you think about making a choice that does not reflect your highest good, take it to the eagle and see your world unfold around that choice.

Stage 12 is a life-long stage where we exist each day, choosing our pure energetic authenticity each moment rather than from what we have been trained to be and trained to think. In this way, we create from beauty and love instead of from fear and control. Stage 12 is the stage of living as a being liberated from patterning, toxins, mood disorders and hang-ups; at stage 12 we have embodied our light, beauty, inner power and peace and can now simply focus on strengthening it. It is only by having done these things that we can perceive through the height and scope of the eagle at all! So it really is a place of honor and great achievement. You have arrived!

At this stage we are doing it all: eating according to the dietary principles, aligning with the breath, practicing our guided meditation daily, challenging our patterns and programming, balancing our inner family, strengthening our flame, attuning ourselves to the highest vibration energy daily and becoming more authentic expressions of love with every day.

At this most sacred stage we become fully aware of how far we have come. We likely see life quite differently. Take a moment to gaze inwardly in your brain and whole body system as well as outwardly above, below and around your energy body at the great benevolent, light force around you. You will have become the thing you gazed upon! You are a living mirror of the golden light you have surrounded yourself with through these practices. You will be walking in your full power, beauty and bliss!

When all stages are complete, allow your body to go through the gentle process of integrating this knowledge and triggering the new energy body awakening at your own pace while you continue to eat, exercise, contemplate and meditate in these ways. Here are a few tips to help you remain in this space until it becomes your natural way of being.

1)   Every time you have a choice – behavioral/response to a thing or person, you can now ask yourself, "Does this resonate with what I now know."

2)   In every choice, instead of thinking what is the right choice or the wrong choice, ask what is the HIGHEST CHOICE.

3)   In order to know whether it is the highest choice you can confirm your decision by asking yourself if the said choice is life-generating or life-depleting.

4)   Remember that just like the cell in your body cannot see your whole body, you cannot see the full scope of what you are really a part of.

5)   Keep in mind that whether it is the foods you eat, the relationships you surround yourself with or the beliefs you hold, if they do not serve the awakening of the new energy body by fanning your electromagnetic firelight then they are depleting you.

PART III
The New Energy Body Integration Plan

CHAPTER NINE
INTEGRATING THE 12-STAGES IN YOUR LIFE

Progressing "stage by stage" <u>in order</u> is essential. The program was created so that each stage builds on the previous knowledge. It's a lot like school. You start at first grade but when you get to fourth grade, you use all the skills you learned in grades 1-3. When you are at stage 4 (embodying your flame) you will be working from a skill set that came from detoxing your diet, guided mediation and proper breathing. By stage 12, you will have acquired a full skill set and be living a life that seamlessly incorporates all that you will have learned.

Start by integrating stages 1-4 in the first month, 5-8 in the second month, 9-12 in the third month and make month four about maintaining all the stages for fully-fledged human empowerment. In some cases it may be better to work even more slowly than this. Listen to yourself and do not feel you need to go quickly. The ability to absorb this material will differ greatly among each person. Enjoy the process and the light that fills you.

What to expect

Allowing yourself to step into the Light means that you will change. In fact, everything in your life will change – your friends, your perceptions, your goals, possibly even your career (or career plan) right down to the structure and dynamics of your closest personal relationships.

When you start to see how your life and choices may have been shrouded in common limitations and see the world through the lens of Light and freedom, you will inevitably find that these new ideas fly in the face of your old carefully guarded concepts (most of which you probably have shared for years and even decades with your nearest and dearest, your community and your personal identity.) Not everyone is going to take well to you coming into your fullness (illuminating all their "comfortable" dark places), including you when you come face-to-face with the things it is time for you to let go of.

While we never wish to deliberately cause discomfort to others, we also cannot deny our growth and be one way in private and hide that Light in public. That is a form of denial that can torment the spirit and hamper your growth. Denial is not the way. I know this because I tried to pretend I was "normal" for years before I stopped trying to hide my true beliefs and interests from my circle of friends, church affiliation, family and clients. I was managing my personality depending on who I was with. In this way, I was rejecting my essence on a very frequent basis. I hated appearing different because it made me feel like I had to protect myself from rejection.

I encountered this first when I started to embrace a clean diet. I had to be discrete in order to avoid the challenging comments and remarks others would make about what seemed at the time a highly unusual way of living; from the from the way I would order in restaurants to the copious amounts of vegetable juice I would drink (not to mention juice fasting, traveling with a juicer and partaking regularly of colonics). I mean who does this stuff!? Well, I did and I do and back then I just didn't want anyone to notice. Even when I had my own practice and became known for this diet lifestyle, I was sensitive to appearing too different. I would always call the waiters around to me so I could quietly give them my order. I never wanted to stand out for being different yet I also didn't want to compromise my great health and energy. Then, when the epiphanies that I discuss in the book awakened me to these non-dietary, equally radical ideas, I felt the dread of having to deal with yet another major thing I thought I would have to be discrete about. It was downright lonely a lot of the time because other than my teacher and two precious friends, I had no one else to share my experiences with (who would understand and support me).

It's all very nice when you get to the stage of having eagle vision. But before that, things can feel quite dark and uncertain (which is work is also known as "the path of the warrior"). Back when I was in the herd, trying to be accepted in the herd while also trying to understand the greater terrain of the jungle and beyond, there was no one to the right or left of me saying, "yes, let's go and look beyond this." It was quite the opposite. I had to come back to my meditation and expansive states of being to be reminded constantly of the illusions all around me in order to keep my focus. The outside world on the streets of Manhattan were brimming with images of materialism, social importance, competition and the like. But the focus paid off and every time I sat with my truth, I could feel my vibrations tingle and rush and I blasted through the programming and it is now completely effortless to be here and see with eagle vision and live with this vaster understanding. Boy, did I ever do the right thing breaking out of the herd! But I didn't know for certain that I would find this state as I was making my break. There was a seed though, a sense that you all have within you that tells you there is something so much more to you than what we see in the herd. Just go with that. Follow that sense inside because it knows where it wants to take you and you can trust it even when it seems scary.

One day I just came on out of the closet for better or worse and some friends did fall by the way side. I had to confront my fears of rejection. But once I did, it wasn't scary. The sub-conscious fears I was walking around with were far more intimidating than the reality. Most of my apprehension turned out to be self-projected. Not much changed other than my perspective of my own public identity. My lesson: one is only vulnerable to judgment if one is judging oneself. If you allow yourself to grow with new ideas, ways of eating and perceiving your world, the world will grow with you. The fear of how other people will react is just another cage we ourselves create, that we can let ourselves out of.

If, in the interim, you find it very challenging to relate with close friends and relatives or feel like you might butt heads with old energy ideas, the best thing to do is simply to soften your heart to all of those around you and to all the issues that may come up in others as well as within yourself. Softening the heart is the way of compassion and it works every time, in every situation.

You see love always overcomes fear and darkness and people will always be softened themselves around a compassionate heart. You'll know you are on the right track if your new outlook makes you more gentle-hearted and compassionate, not less so; more generous of spirit and understanding, not less so.

If, it happens that your change attracts conflict after conflict, you might take an honest look at yourself to see if you are engaging in judgment and bringing old energy ways of relating to spirituality like dogma and preaching into your energy body – either consciously or subconsciously. As disconnected as the modern human has become, he can still almost always pick up the "vibe" you are broadcasting. People generally can feel what you are putting out even if they only sense it subconsciously and their reaction to it is subconscious even though it may manifest materially. Light and knowledge, while first for your own growth, is ultimately for humanity and all the earth. It's not about becoming better than someone else. All your growth is ultimately for the for the group's glory (mankind, earth-kind and ultimately, "cosmic-kind") – not the individual (which was the old energy way). People will sense when your actions are selfish and when they are self-less.

The underlying thread that we would be foolish to forget even for a moment is that we are all deeply interconnected. Our ego can get caught up in the power that this knowledge brings – you become enriched with bliss, empowered by knowing what you are and what your ultimate enfoldment will mean, you will become more radiant, beautiful, eloquent, perceptive, intelligent and so much more.

On the other hand, as much as the Light gifts us with empowerment, it also reveals all our dark corners and corridors. This is not an appealing concept to those who cling to their egos because to let go and let the Light in is all but impossible without the depth of surrender that comes from unconditional acceptance of the entire self – not just the self that appears to be strong and successful. Further, once the love Light starts to enter the body, it cannot help but begin to heal the pain that has created the need to dominate in the first place. So you see, **there is nothing to fear when the Light comes through you** – from yourself or the rest of the awakening world because Light is knowledge and the ultimate knowledge is Love which trumps all things.

You might be asking yourself, how will I be able to gauge my progress? How will I know that my New Energy Body is awakening and that my 12 strand DNA has been activated? Well, the awakening will come in stages that may be imperceptible at times and more obvious at other times.

A good way to gage your progress is to notice if you are gaining more perception from your experiences and feeling less disturbed by the dramas around you. When conflict arises are you taking the lessons and growing? Responding in your higher truth rather than reacting in your old ways? If so, this is a major accomplishment and a great indicator of your progress.

However, while overall there will be increasing harmony in all areas of your life, know that there may also be difficult trials when you are in the process of taking your greatest leaps. In this way, one should not rely on serenity as the sole indicator of growth.

One thing to be aware of is a growing sense of feeling yourself as a part of the greater body of life. You will have access to more than just your identity consciousness as you grow – you will have access to global consciousness and planetary consciousness. This will come up as feelings, thoughts, ideas, information that comes through at dreamtime and surprisingly enlightened perspectives that take the place of old ones as you allow yourself to expand and feel yourself as one with the greater whole.

The distinct changes in your consciousness should feel very comfortable and familiar. You may even start to tap into sensations of moving through the worlds. For example, you may feel your awareness expand to link up to the universe and Source light and then contract back to feel fully "in your body." You might even be able to tap into the sensation of contracting into the space of an atom and yet feeling the vastness of space within that atom. This is not essential for growth but it is an indication that your consciousness is fluid and you are seeing yourself as being more than just your body. You are feeling your essence and knowing yourself as that limitless essence.

Most importantly though, you will come to know in your heart that you are "Light of the One Light" and that This great Source Light dwells in you just as you dwell in It. You will embody the sentiment of such expressions as, "You are He that sent you," and "I am that I Am."

You will remember. That's the best way to tell. You will remember (in ways that the left brain may not be adept at down-stepping into words) who you are and the limitlessness you are connected with. You will experience an undeniable remembering – as though you are waking up from a dream.

I am honored to share this with you.

Yours in the most joyful service,

Natalia

For more information about Natalia Rose please visit: Therawfooddetoxdiet.com
The Rose Program, LLC
New York, New York
Contact: Natalia@therawfooddetoxdiet.com
Phone: (212) 752-6458

Made in the USA
Lexington, KY
27 July 2013